Diabetes: a guide to patient management for practice nurses

Diabetes: a guide to patient management for practice nurses

JENNIFER FARR

AND

MAGGIE WATKINSON

RADCLIFFE MEDICAL PRESS
OXFORD

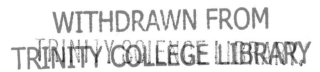

© 1989 Radcliffe Medical Press Ltd
15 Kings Meadow, Ferry Hinksey Road, Oxford OX2 0DP

British Library Cataloguing in Publication Data

Farr, Jennifer
Diabetes: a guide to patient management for practice nurses
1. Diabetic patients. Nursing
I. Title   II. Watkinson, Margaret Anne
610.73'69

ISBN 1 870905 31 8

Printed and bound in Great Britain
Typeset by Advance Typesetting, Oxfordshire

Contents

Foreword

ONE of the major advances over the last ten years has been the improved care offered to people with diabetes by the primary health care team. An increasing number of general practitioners have become involved in shared care schemes with the local hospital with some organizing diabetic mini clinics within the surgery. This has inevitably meant that many practice nurses have become involved in diabetes care, being asked to assist in the mini clinic and to educate the patients. It has proved quite daunting to some practice nurses whose only experience in caring for diabetic patients has been during their general training which in some cases may have been a considerable number of years ago.

I wish this excellent book, which is aimed at nurses working in general practice, had been available ten years ago when I began caring for people with diabetes. It covers every aspect of patient care, the text is down-to-earth, explaining everything carefully and clearly, guiding the reader step-by-step from diagnosis through to treatment and, most importantly, patient education.

I am sure everyone who reads this book will do so with enjoyment and at the same time profit from the valuable information gained. It will be invaluable as a reference book and be of benefit not only to practice nurses but to every other member of the primary health care team helping to educate them in this most interesting and rewarding area of nursing.

Elvia Steward
Practice Sister/Diabetes Specialist Nurse
Kings Lynn, Norfolk

Preface

GENERAL practice provides the ideal setting in which to care for patients with diabetes mellitus. A team approach and continuity of care are essential ingredients for effective management which must enable the patient to learn self care and to take responsibility for their own disease.

The practice nurse is a key figure in the practice team and it is she who will see the patient most frequently and who will be charged with their education and be responsible for ensuring that they are monitoring and treating their diabetes effectively.

This book is written for the practice nurse. Not only does it provide her with the necessary background information on the disease, its possible complications and how to prevent them to help her to educate the patient, but it also makes suggestions on *how* to develop, implement and evaluate an educational programme, while stressing the importance of involving the patient in the learning process.

The way in which diabetic care is organized in general practice varies considerably from those practices which see their diabetic patients on an *ad hoc* basis or those who provide protected time in ordinary surgeries, to those who run well-structured diabetic mini clinics. This book discusses the advantages and disadvantages of each system and gives suggestions on how to overcome what may seem daunting barriers to setting up an organized system of care.

Jennifer Farr
Maggie Watkinson
November 1989

Acknowledgements

THE authors would like to thank Laurie King, Chiropodist and Jane Porteous, Dietician for their contributions to the book.

Help and advice was also given by

Dr Jane Smith, Ophthalmologist, Oxford Eye Hospital
Dr Peter Tasker, General Practitioner, Kings Lynn
Dr Tony Knight, Consultant, Stoke Mandeville Hospital, Aylesbury
Dr Steve O'Rahilly
Constance Martin, Practice Nurse, Eastbourne

Thanks also to Gillian Nineham and Kate Martin at Radcliffe Medical Press and to Peter, Ben and Gareth.

The Publishers would like to thank Boehringer Corporation (London) Ltd without whose considerable financial help publication would not have been possible.

CHAPTER 1

What is diabetes?

DIABETES mellitus is a common chronic condition affecting 1–2% of the population. There is probably one undiagnosed patient in the community for every one diagnosed.

Non-insulin-dependent diabetes mellitus (NIDDM)

The prevalence of known maturity onset diabetes mellitus, Type II or NIDDM is around 1% of the population in the UK. It usually affects people from middle age onwards and women more commonly than men. In many cases it is associated with obesity and may be precipitated by the use of drugs such as steroids and diuretics. There is some familial tendency.

Blood insulin levels can initially be high in NIDDM patients as the pancreas produces extra insulin to compensate for the deficient working of the cells' insulin receptors. Patients who are overweight may have too few of these receptors; in other patients their receptors may not be functioning for some reason. The pancreas therefore increases its production of insulin in an effort to allow the cell to take in sugar, eventually it becomes partially exhausted and stops working to full capacity.

Initially, NIDDM can often be treated by diet alone, but later it may be necessary to introduce hypoglycaemic drugs as well. Some NIDDM patients eventually need insulin if diet and tablets fail to achieve satisfactory control. They are then known as insulin-treated diabetics and not insulin-dependent diabetics. There is a significant difference between these two terms (*see* page 3 for classification).

Aetiology

There are certain factors which predispose to NIDDM.

Age – It would seem that during the ageing process, glucose metabolism becomes less efficient. This is known as impaired glucose tolerance but someone with impaired glucose tolerance does not necessarily have diabetes (*see* page 5 on glucose tolerance tests).

There are two schools of thought about the effect of deficient glucose metabolism in the elderly. Some research has shown that a 70-year-old with diabetes mellitus may have a reduced chance of surviving the next decade due to coronary vascular disease resulting from moderately raised blood glucose levels. Other research has shown that diabetes mellitus in the elderly has little or no effect on longevity.

Obesity – NIDDM is more common in the obese than those of normal weight. The obese tend to have a reduced number of cell receptors for insulin which results in impaired glucose tolerance.

Hyperglycaemia – When insulin resistance is present as a result of obesity, the beta cells secrete increased amounts of insulin in order to maintain normal glucose levels. If more pressure is put on these already overworked beta cells (e.g. illness, high carbohydrate (CHO) diet) a further weight gain will result in increased blood glucose levels and beta cell function will deteriorate further.

Racial difference – The prevalence of NIDDM varies with race. In Western Europe it is 1–2% of the population. North American Pima Indians have a 35–40% prevalence. The main reason for this is their genetic predisposition which is increased by in-breeding. An additional factor is probably environmental with their transition from a low calorie diet and a high level of exercise to a much more sedentary lifestyle and Western food products. The effect of diet and lifestyle is also highlighted by the fact that there is a higher prevalence of NIDDM in Asians living in Britain than in those living on the Asian continent.

Genetics – There is a familial tendency to inherit diabetes, especially NIDDM. If one identical twin has this form of the disease the other will invariably develop it eventually. If the patient has NIDDM, 25% of their first degree relatives will develop it (parents, siblings, children). If two NIDDM patients have a child, that child will have a 1:10 chance of developing it. If one parent has NIDDM the risk is 1:60.

Insulin-dependent diabetes mellitus (IDDM)

Insulin-dependent diabetes mellitus (IDDM) has also been known as juvenile onset or Type I diabetes, but the most up-to-date classification is IDDM.

Approximately 10–15% of all diabetics are insulin-dependent, and require injected insulin to live. This is because the islets of Langerhans fail and are unable to produce any, or only a very small amount of insulin.

IDDM usually affects people under forty who are thin or of normal weight. The onset of the condition is rapid, over a few days or weeks, and the patient presents with weight loss, polyuria, polydipsia and lethargy. The patient will also have glycosuria and hyperglycaemia, and is likely to be dehydrated. Other conditions which might be present are pruritus vulvae, balanitis and other local infections such as boils or cellulitis. Some patients will present in ketoacidosis, with varying degrees of severity.

Aetiology

The genetic make-up of an individual will have some bearing on whether or not they develop insulin-dependent diabetes. Research has shown that individuals with certain inherited antigens have increased susceptibility. In order for them to go on to develop IDDM, it is thought that there is an environmental 'trigger'. Current thinking is that viruses may be responsible but the evidence is unclear. It has been noted that there are more insulin-dependent diabetics diagnosed in the winter months, possibly due to the increase in viral infections at this time of year.

Classification of diabetes mellitus

Although this table is only a rough guide, it is useful for patient management. It is important to be aware that patients may have features from both lists.

Table 1.1 Classification of diabetes mellitus

IDDM	NIDDM
Insulin-dependent	Non-insulin-dependent
	Not normally insulin requiring/sometimes insulin treated
Usually under 40 at diagnosis	Usually over 40 at diagnosis
Ketotic prone	Non-ketotic
Thin	Overweight
Rapid presentation	Slow onset
Family history less common	Family history common
Often winter presentation – ?due to viral infection	No seasonal presentation

Types of secondary diabetes

These are uncommon, however they can be caused by the following factors.

Insulin antagonists

An excess of endocrine hormones can cause secondary diabetes. In acromegaly there is an excess of growth hormone; in Cushing's syndrome an excess of cortisol; in phaeochromocytoma an excess of catecholamines – adrenaline and noradrenaline. All these hormones are antagonistic to insulin, thereby reducing its effectiveness and often resulting in diabetes. Insulin is not usually required for its treatment.

Chronic pancreatitis, cancer of the pancreas and surgical removal of the pancreas

These conditions can cause raised blood glucose levels, and thus diabetes.

Haemochromotosis

This destroys the function of beta cells due to iron deposits in the pancreas.

Corticosteroid therapy

This therapy causes impaired glucose tolerance or frank diabetes.

Diuretics

Diuretics e.g. bendrofluazide, frusemide can be the 'final insult' and cause increased glucose intolerance.

The contraceptive pill

Use of the contraceptive pill can result in impaired glucose tolerance.

There are also around 30 rare genetic disorders associated with diabetes mellitus.

CHAPTER 2

Diagnosis

THE World Health Organisation (WHO) and the National Diabetes Data Group in the United States specify criteria for diagnosis. The presence of symptoms such as thirst, polyuria, glycosuria and weight loss plus a random blood glucose greater than 11 mmol/l or macrovascular disease and/or retinopathy would confirm diagnosis. For those with blood glucose levels near normal or just above the WHO criteria, a glucose tolerance test can confirm diagnosis.

Glucose tolerance test (GTT)

Table 2.1	Fasting	Two hour post glucose
Normal		
Venous whole blood	<6.7 mmol/l	<6.7 mmol/l
Capillary whole blood	<6.7 mmol/l	<7.8 mmol/l
Venous plasma	<7.8 mmol/l	<7.8 mmol/l
Impaired Glucose Tolerance		
Venous whole blood	<6.7 mmol/l	6.7–10.0 mmol/l
Capillary whole blood	<6.7 mmol/l	7.8–11.1 mmol/l
Venous plasma	<7.8 mmol/l	7.8–11.1 mmol/l
Diabetes Mellitus		
Venous whole blood	≥6.7 mmol/l	≥10.0 mmol/l
Capillary whole blood	≥6.7 mmol/l	≥11.1 mmol/l
Venous plasma	≥7.8 mmol/l	≥11.1 mmol/l

(The World Health Organisation guidelines on Oral Glucose Tolerance Test 1985.)

A normal value is cited as a fasting venous blood glucose and two hours post glucose load value of less than 6.7 mmol/l.

Fasting venous and capillary whole blood glucose levels of ≥6.7 mmol/l or fasting venous plasma levels of ≥7.8 mmol/l are considered diagnostic of diabetes mellitus. A glucose load is then given and a two hour post glucose value of ≥10 mmol/l for venous whole blood and ≥11.1 for capillary whole blood confirm the diagnosis.

Any intermediate values or combination of intermediate values can be defined as impaired glucose tolerance.

The confirmation of diabetes should not be taken lightly as the repercussions on life insurance, driving, employment etc may be serious. Impaired glucose tolerance is not 'diabetes' but does have a high morbidity and mortality rate due to macrovascular disease.

Consideration should be given as to who should receive the test. It is well known that in the elderly a slightly raised result from a glucose tolerance test would not be considered abnormal, but it would be in a pregnant woman or a young person.

Those who show glycosuria but normal blood glucose levels should be informed of this, told they are not diabetic and documented.

Protocol for glucose tolerance test

- Eat normally up to overnight fast
- Fast overnight
- Patient should rest and not smoke
- Fasting blood glucose test taken
- 75g of diluted glucose is drunk in 250–350 ml water. Blood is then taken at 30 minute intervals

An alternative method is a blood glucose level tested one hour and two hours after glucose is taken.

Urine may also be tested at hourly intervals for two to two and a half hours at the same time as GTT.

Diagnosing diabetes in patients without acute symptoms

The acute symptoms of diabetes mellitus are weight loss, thirst, polyuria and weakness and lethargy. Diagnosing patients with these symptoms as diabetic is relatively straightforward. However, there are other signs and symptoms which may suggest to the nurse that the patient has glucose levels which are higher than normal.

- Balanitis/pruritus vulvae
- Sugar deposits from urine splashes on shoes (men)
- Blurred vision due to hyperglycaemia, cataract or diabetic retinopathy following years of undiagnosed diabetes
- Leg and foot ulcers
- Peripheral vascular disease
- Boils, carbuncles and infections
- Family history

Remember that some diabetics may have few or none of these symptoms.

Patients may be identified by routine urine testing on admission to hospital, in occupational health checks, MOTs, Well Man or Woman clinics, antenatal clinics, etc. Urinalysis does not always reflect raised blood glucose levels however, particularly in patients with high renal thresholds (*see* pages 11–12).

Social and psychological problems following diagnosis

In a newly diagnosed diabetic there are typically five stages through which they have to pass to reach acceptance of their disease. This is known as the grieving process. The stages are shock, denial, anger, depression and acceptance. The diagnosis of a chronic disease gives the sufferer a great sense of personal loss and it can feel as if part of them has died.

To achieve a healthy state of acceptance the whole grieving process needs to be completed. Often this does not happen and the patient remains at the stage of anger or denial. This is particularly so in young adults who may rebel against their diabetes. The pubescent adolescent already experiencing stress from the changes taking place in relationships, from peer group pressure, and the move from school to work or university does not easily accept the fact that they have a chronic disease. The diabetes may be ignored and neglected. These patients have special needs and the practice nurse is in an ideal position to address them.

Diagnosis in later life is usually more easily accepted. After the initial shock patients tend to be more philosophical about it. They are often resigned to the fact that illness is more likely to strike as they get older. However, there can be exceptions and some older patients are devastated by the news.

Simple comments can give considerable insight into how patients feel about their disease.

A 42-year-old female school teacher:
'I felt immortal and couldn't believe that I would ever have a chronic disease. My body has failed me. What will fail next?'

A 23-year-old student:
'If I do as little as possible to look after my diabetes, and just take my insulin, then I don't have to remind myself too often I have diabetes.'

A 35-year-old pub landlady:
'I tend to my diet occasionally. I do blood tests and of course I take my insulin, but it's not *my* diabetes, it's someone else's!'

Until the patient has accepted their disease, compliance can be a problem. The most constructive action practice nurses can take is to support the patient through this period and remember that 'nagging' produces more guilt and resentment. If blood glucose control is very unsatisfactory, small goals can be set over a long period of time, for example from no blood testing at all to testing once a week.

In some cases there may not be any improvement in attitude and control and the nurse has to accept that she has informed the patient of the risks they run if their diabetes is not controlled, and that she must now stand by to support if necessary and be available in times of crisis.

Other psychological problems experienced by patients are low self-esteem; feeling like a second class citizen; feeling a freak and not liking the injections because of the association of needles with drug abuse. Some patients are so frightened of hypoglycaemic attacks that they maintain their blood glucose at higher than normal levels in order to avoid them. Depression may result from anxiety about diabetic complications, disability or early death. Occasionally a patient will use their diabetes to manipulate those around them, inducing hypoglycaemia or becoming hyperglycaemic by altering their eating patterns or reducing insulin. This behaviour usually begins in childhood and becomes a habit to attract attention or allow them to avoid a situation they would rather not confront.

The practice nurse is likely to be more involved in the care of newly diagnosed NIDDs than IDDs, and although NIDDM may not appear to have as dramatic an effect on the patient's life as IDDM, the patient will still have many fears and questions. Initially they will want to know what diabetes is and how the treatment will affect them; they will want reassurance that they can continue to lead a normal life and that well controlled diabetes will reduce the risk of complications. They will want to know how their diabetes will affect their job and career, whether they can drive, how they will need to adapt their lifestyle and whether they can have children.

Patients need support, particularly at the time of diagnosis, but this support needs to be continued even when the patient has settled into a routine. It is up to the nurse and doctor to recognize when this support is needed.

CHAPTER 3

Monitoring for the non-insulin-dependent diabetic

MONITORING is essential for all diabetics, and one of the practice nurse's major roles is to ensure that the patient can demonstrate proficiency in monitoring, interpret the results and understand their implications.

An awareness of the reasons for regular monitoring and problems that can arise from poor control is important as is an ability to recognize the features of hypo- and hyperglycaemia.

Blood glucose monitoring

Almost all IDDs should monitor their blood glucose levels, and it is useful in NIDDs as it aids patient compliance and understanding of their disease and enables them to seek prompt medical advice when hypo- or hyperglycaemia occurs.

There are some NIDDs who will particularly benefit from blood glucose monitoring:

- those with gestational diabetes;
- those who are poorly controlled and may need insulin treatment;
- those who experience frequent hypoglycaemic episodes whilst on tablets;
- those with a high or low renal threshold;
- those trying to conceive: levels should be in the range 4–8 mmol/l for 2–3 months prior to conception;
- those who are pregnant: good control can reduce the risk of miscarriage and foetal abnormalities.

(Further details on blood glucose monitoring will be found in Chapter 4.)

Urine testing

Most NIDDs monitor control of their disease by urine testing. Urine testing may be useful for the elderly in particular, for whom blood glucose monitoring is not always possible due to poor eyesight or poor manual dexterity. Other patients may refuse to monitor their blood glucose because they have needle phobia, do not think it is necessary or find the technique too difficult and cannot provide reliable results. This is often due to lack of understanding and the practice nurse has a role to play here in educating the patient.

It is important to explain to the patient why monitoring glucose levels is so important. Obviously you need to decide how much detail to go into on an individual basis, depending on the ability and willingness of the patient to absorb the information.

It is advisable for urine to be tested frequently, particularly when first diagnosed and during treatment changes. The first morning urine sample should be used and then the urine tested two hours after each meal.

Glucose in the urine in the first test of the morning indicates poor glycaemic control and a fasting blood glucose of more than 6.7 mmol/l will confirm this.

The first test of the day should be on the specimen passed on rising. This helps to discover if blood glucose levels peaked during the night, i.e. since the bladder was last emptied although it will *not* show if a hypoglycaemic attack occurred in the night. In other words, this retrospective testing is looking at glycaemic control through the 'eyes of the kidney'.

Both nurse and patient should be aware that although constant negative results may reflect good glycaemic control, they may also indicate hypoglycaemic or near hypoglycaemic levels. If this is the case the oral hypoglycaemic therapy should be reviewed and reduced.

Urine can also be tested to detect post-prandial glucose peaks. The bladder should be emptied before meal times and the first urine specimen, passed one or two hours after the meal, should be tested. An alternative form of testing is that the bladder is emptied approximately 30 minutes before a meal and then a sample is tested just before eating. This shows a 'here and now' urine glucose. A pre-prandial test showing glucose present will indicate that the post-prandial result will be even higher.

Initial testing following diagnosis should be done more frequently, i.e. four times a day, eventually reducing the frequency as a majority of negative results are obtained.

The testing regimen should show a cross-section of the results taken during the week at different times (*see* Table 3.1). Rotate the times to show whether there is glycosuria at any time of day.

Table 3.1 A cross-section of urine testing at different times over a week.

Date	Before Breakfast	After Breakfast	Before Midday Meal	After Midday Meal	Before Evening Meal	After Evening Meal
1.6.89	0%					
2.6.89		¼%				
3.6.89				2%		
4.6.89						1%
5.6.89	0%					
6.6.89		½%				
7.6.89				1%		
8.6.89						0%

Record keeping is important for the patient's own information and should be shown to any health professional who asks to see it.

Remember: more frequent testing is needed when ill (*see* p. 62, Chapter 8).

The mechanism of glycosuria

Glucose is freely filtered by the glomerulus and is present in the filtrate at the same concentration as in the blood. At the proximal tubule glucose is reabsorbed. The amount of glucose which is reabsorbed is limited. Once the blood glucose levels climb beyond around 10 mmol/l, glucose appears in the urine. This is known as the renal threshold. Thereafter the degree of glycosuria increases in proportion to the amount of glucose in the blood.

A simple way to explain this to a patient is to use the 'dam analogy' below.

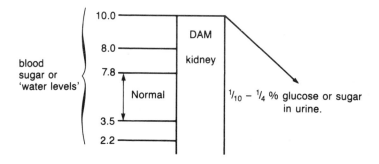

Figure 3.1 The dam analogy.

Glucose spills out of the urine as though the kidney is a dam and cannot hold back the glucose in the blood as the levels rise.

Patients need to understand the principle of the renal threshold for glucose and those with normal thresholds should aim to have glucose-free urine at all times. Account needs to be taken of those with a high or a low renal threshold.

Low renal threshold Patients are said to have a low renal threshold when glucose shows in their urine while their blood glucose level is below 10 mmol/l. A low threshold can occur during pregnancy.

Some patients with glycosuria may be wrongly diagnosed as having diabetes, so it is important to perform a blood glucose test as confirmation. Glycosuria can occur as a result of renal disease and so this should be ruled out. (*see* section on glucose tolerance testing, page 5.)

High renal threshold Patients have a high renal threshold when glucose does not appear in the urine although the blood glucose level is more than 10 mmol/l. In some elderly people the blood glucose level may be as high as 17 mmol/l before glycosuria occurs. Again blood glucose testing is essential.

Problems with urine testing

Patients do not usually experience problems with technique in urine testing as they can with blood testing.

However, problems with urine testing may arise in patients with low or high renal thresholds for glucose. Those with low renal thresholds can become hypoglycaemic in trying to achieve negative results and those with high renal thresholds can achieve negative results when dietary indiscretions have been committed. This latter problem is compounded in the elderly as the renal threshold rises as part of the ageing process. Any abnormal renal threshold should be recorded, the patient made aware of it, and advised to monitor their blood glucose as well as their urine.

Sometimes patients are not able to co-operate or are unable to test their blood. This means it is difficult to detect the pattern of poor glycaemic control and therefore difficult to know how to change therapy. One solution is to work in conjunction with the diabetes specialist nurse and district nurse and organize blood and urine testing at home for a couple of weeks. During this period you can compare urine test levels with blood glucose levels and work out the renal threshold and then alter the hypoglycaemic agents or transfer the patient to insulin. To do this accurately, ask the patient for a double voided urine specimen and measure their blood glucose at the same time. The patient should then have a better idea of what the urine tests mean in relation to satisfactory blood glucose control.

CHAPTER 4

Monitoring for the insulin-dependent diabetic

ALL diabetic patients should monitor their metabolic control, to enable them to manage it themselves or to provide their professional carers or relatives with the information to do it for them.

Most patients taking insulin should monitor their blood glucose levels rather than performing urinalysis, but some are unwilling or unable to do it. The accurate results and strict monitoring obtainable from blood glucose testing are not essential in the very elderly. However, some elderly patients may find it difficult to provide the double voided urine specimens required for accurate urinalysis.

Insulin doses can be changed according to urinary glucose results, but they should be interpreted with caution as they do not always reflect blood glucose concentrations. This is because of individual variations in renal thresholds and differences in the levels of blood glucose which cause levels of glycosuria to increase. A further problem is that, assuming a patient's renal threshold is 10 mmol/l, a negative urine result can mean that the individual is hypoglycaemic, normal or slightly hyperglycaemic.

Why monitor

Monitoring blood and/or urine provides accurate information to enable diabetes to be managed and treated on a day-to-day basis including the adjustment of diet, exercise and insulin. Improved control on a daily basis leads to improved control over a long period of time, and it is hoped, to a reduction in long term complications or at least a delay in their onset and severity.

The ability to control blood glucose levels should lead to an improved knowledge base. The patient may learn how certain situations, such as heavy exercise periods, alter his or her blood glucose level and how to deal with similar situations subsequently. Another advantage is that many patients find that they are more motivated to manage their diabetes and develop confidence in themselves, both as a person and as a 'diabetic'.

Those patients who develop hypo- and hyperglycaemia rapidly will be warned by monitoring their blood glucose levels and be able to take relevant action and avert emergency situations.

While educating the patient about monitoring, other topics related to diabetes will inevitably arise and the nurse can use these opportunities constructively to improve the patient's overall knowledge.

Those contemplating pregnancy, or who are already pregnant, whether or not they are treated with insulin, should perform blood glucose monitoring to ensure that their diabetes is exceptionally well controlled. Most women are well motivated during this period.

When to monitor

Advice on how frequently to monitor varies from District to District and the practice nurse should check local protocol. It may vary from twice every day to four times a day, twice a week. In Oxford patients are advised to monitor at least once daily, at different times of the day. For patients using blood glucose monitoring the tests should be performed before main meals and just before the bedtime snack (Table 4.1).

Table 4.1

Date	Before Breakfast	Before Midday meal	Before Evening meal	Before Bedtime
1.6.89	X			
2.6.89		X		
3.6.89			X	
4.6.89				X
5.6.89	X			
6.6.89		X		
7.6.89			X	
8.6.89				X

The results can also be plotted on a graph. These are provided in most of the record books supplied by commercial companies. Charting results in this way can make it easier to identify blood glucose levels which are too high or low at certain times of the day.

Once-daily testing is sufficient if the diabetes is generally well controlled. The number of tests should be increased to at least four times a day (before main meals and at bedtime) at times of 'unstable diabetes', that is at diagnosis and in the immediate period thereafter, in stressful situations and during illness and pregnancy (Table 4.2).

Table 4.2

Date	Before Breakfast	Before Midday meal	Before Evening meal	Before Bedtime
1.6.89	X	X	X	X

Another regimen, testing four times a day, twice a week is shown in Table 4.3.

Table 4.3

Date	Before Breakfast	Before Midday meal	Before Evening meal	Before Bedtime
1.6.89	X	X	X	X
6.6.89	X	X	X	X

If they use the regimen shown in Table 4.3, patients should ensure that they choose one working day and one 'rest' day as there may be marked differences in results due to the amount of exercise taken. Some patients prefer this method because they find it difficult to remember to do their testing using a once-daily regimen. The disadvantage is that they do not have any idea of what their blood glucose levels are on the five days on which they do not monitor.

It is often recommended that pregnant women with diabetes monitor seven times a day for the whole of the pregnancy (*see* Table 4.4).

Table 4.4

Date	Before B'fast	After B'fast	Before M meal	After M meal	Before E meal	After E meal	Before Bedtime
1.6.89	X	X	X	X	X	X	X
2.6.89	X	X	X	X	X	X	X

This enables them to adjust their insulin doses to ensure normo-glycaemia throughout the day.

Those on multiple insulin regimens such as Ultratard and Actrapid via the Novopen are advised to test more frequently to allow them to achieve greater flexibility by altering the carbohydrate content and timing of their meals. These regimens tend to be used mainly for the younger diabetic. Sometimes these patients are also advised to test post-prandial blood glucose levels to get accurate profiles over a 24-hour period.

It is important that patients understand the importance of monitoring regularly and that they persevere. When the diabetes is well controlled for a period of time, there may be a tendency to allow the frequency of measurements to fall and this can lead to poorer control.

Insulin-treated patients testing their urine may perform tests following the profiles shown in Tables 4.1 and 4.2. They should also follow the same guidelines as those performing blood glucose monitoring with regard to the frequency of measurements.

How to monitor

There are various blood glucose monitoring strips available, most of which can be obtained on prescription. Most of them utilize a reaction between glucose and chemicals impregnated on pads on the end of the strip. The pads change colour according to the amount of glucose in the blood. The strips are all used in slightly different ways and it is important that the manufacturer's instructions are carried out explicitly.

Full details can be obtained from the companies concerned. It is advisable for each practice to use one system to enable them to become proficient. It should be borne in mind however that individual patients may be using different techniques.

All the systems require the strips to be well covered in blood and this can be a problem for some patients. The skin must be cleaned before the finger is pricked to avoid accidental contamination from sweet substances which may be present. To help improve blood flow the patient should wash his or her hands in warm water or swing the arm vigorously for one minute. The best fingers to use are the third and fourth fingers as the skin is often softer and less thick. The pulp at the top of the finger is sometimes used but this may be painful and bruising may occur. For people such as typists or braille readers who use the tips of their fingers, the pulp should be avoided. The side of the end of the finger is the preferred site for lancing.

Patients should prick their fingers using a lancet, with or without a device designed specifically for the purpose. There are a variety of these available for purchase by the patient, and they are generally inexpensive. Most of the lancets are available on prescription and different brands are on the whole not interchangeable. They should only be used once, but the base plates or platforms may be washed and used again.

When the skin has been pierced, the drop of blood should be allowed to hang on the end of the finger as all the systems require that only blood is placed on the strip, without the skin coming into contact with it (see Fig. 4.1).

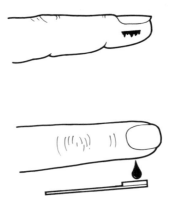

Figure 4.1.

The pads on the strips are designed to 'draw out' the drop to ensure that it covers the total surface. The blood should not be spread over the pad using the finger. Squeezing the finger at the top will suppress blood flow. 'Milking' the finger from the base will elicit a good sized drop.

If an adequate drop of blood cannot be obtained, it is probably better not to perform the test as inaccuracies may result in inappropriate action being taken.

Once the blood has been placed on the strip it is extremely important that the timing is adhered to accurately with strict reference to the manufacturer's instructions.

Following wiping and colour development time the strip is compared with the scale on the side of the container. It is important that the comparison is made in good light to ensure that the reading is accurate. With practice patients and staff can make satisfactory estimations of blood glucose results reading the strips visually. Making a 'guesstimate' if the results fall clearly between two of the zones on the container should be actively encouraged as otherwise there may be a tendency to round them down.

Some patients new to blood glucose monitoring are not confident about their ability to read strips accurately. With some systems they can store used strips in an empty container, with the lid fastened securely, and return them to the practice nurse for her to check the results. The date and time of the test can be recorded on the back of the strip.

The results should be recorded: most of the commercial companies provide record sheets or monitoring diaries, with space for notes.

Meters

Results obtained with correctly used meters compare favourably with laboratory results and some health professionals feel that patients should use meters to enable them to obtain more accurate blood glucose results. There are, however, disadvantages to using meters. Many patients cannot afford them. There is also a tendency to rely implicitly on technology and assume that machines are better, but more can go wrong using a meter than doing blood glucose measurements by eye. However, patients with colour blindness or poor eyesight may retain their independence by using a meter. For those who are totally blind a talking meter is available. Many patients prefer to use a meter, and for those who need to achieve excellent control, such as pregnant women, a meter may be preferable.

Results and action

Desirable blood glucose levels should ideally be within the normoglycaemic range to prevent short and long term complications, but there are many other factors to be considered. The age, state of health and quality of life of the patient need to be taken into account. Their motivation and intellectual and physical abilities are also relevant. For each individual there should be an acceptable range of blood glucose levels developed according to these factors.

Good control is generally deemed to be blood glucose levels of 3–8 mmol/l, and patients should be advised to try to achieve levels of 3.5–6.5 mmol/l before main meals and bed. Adjusting insulin doses and diet to achieve these levels can be undertaken by most patients following advice and given support while they are learning. There are certain principles to be followed. Change in diet and insulin dose adjustment should not be undertaken at the same time because confusion will arise as it will not be known which change has had the effect. It is generally better to start with simple measures. For example, moving 10 g of carbohydrate from one meal to another may solve fluctuating blood glucose levels without changing insulin doses. It may also be that overall control is improved with dietary measures alone. Before patients and staff start to adjust insulin doses they need to know the timing profiles of each one, bearing in mind that these will be slightly different for each individual patient. When insulins are adjusted, only one at a time should be altered, and it is best to start with the evening longer acting insulin if the blood glucose levels are raised overall, to achieve a normal blood glucose before breakfast. The next one to adjust should be the longer acting insulin given before breakfast which will affect the blood glucose before the evening meal. Once these are satisfactory the short acting insulins which affect the pre-lunch and bedtime blood glucose levels may be adjusted (*see* Table 4.5).

Table 4.5

Insulin	Time given	Which reading affected
Longer acting	Before evening meal	Pre-breakfast
Longer acting	Before breakfast	Pre-evening meal
Short acting	Before breakfast	Pre-lunch
Short acting	Before evening meal	Bedtime

If blood glucose levels are high or low at one time of day, the appropriate insulin only needs to be altered.

Insulin doses should be changed by 2–4 units at a time; this is usually sufficient to effect the desired result. It is advisable to monitor the effects of a change before altering another insulin and not to change more than one insulin dose in a 24-hour period. Patients who are using long acting insulins such as Ultratard should be advised not to change this more often than every three days as it will take that long for the effect to become apparent.

HbA$_1$

Glycosylated or glycated haemoglobin measurement is often used to assess long term control. As each new red blood cell is made, a chemical reaction takes place between glucose and part of the haemoglobin molecule. This fraction is called HbA$_1$. The amount of glucose that 'sticks' is in direct proportion to the amount present in the blood. As a red blood cell lasts 120 days, in any one sample there will be old and new cells, and the result will give an indication of control over the preceding six to eight weeks. The amount of glycosylated haemoglobin is expressed as a percentage of the total; the upper limit of normal in most laboratories is between 8 and 9% and control is deemed to be very poor if the level is 12% or above.

Fructosamine

Another way of assessing long term control is to measure fructosamine. This is made up of glycated plasma proteins, mostly albumin. It is a cheaper method than glycosylated haemoglobin as the process can be automated. The result is influenced by serum albumin concentrations and plasma protein half lives and is difficult to standardize. The result will give an indication of control over the preceding two to four weeks and is most useful in pregnancy.

CHAPTER 5

Education of the diabetic patient

THE main goal in educating diabetic patients is to help them to achieve self care and involve them and their families and friends actively in the control of the disease and the prevention of complications. The approach needs to be a holistic one with a learning programme devised for each individual patient, and in general practice it is the nurse who is ideally suited to the role of educator and to providing continuity of care. While the patient is accepting and adapting to his condition, the nurse can build up a relationship of mutual trust and respect and provide support. She can begin to prepare him for the future and introduce him to other diabetics and the local branch of the British Diabetic Association (BDA).

Self care

The emphasis in self care is on health promotion rather than illness. Individuals have a responsibility for their own health and they have a right to choose the actions they take to achieve and maintain it. Some patients do not want or are unable to accept this responsibility. Some health professionals may find it difficult to allow the patient the freedom to exercise his right to choose when they have been used to the patient depending on them.

Partnership with patients

Traditionally nurses have felt that patients should accept their advice because they have knowledge and skills related to health care as a result of their training and experience. Nurses did things to and for the patient, and made decisions for them. This relationship was one of caring for and could be likened to mothering. It fostered dependence and allowed little opportunity for growth of the individual patient as a person. Partnership involves the patient making his contribution to the care; they are after all the expert on what their needs as an individual are. This relationship is an equal and adult one in which the patient develops by using the nurse's knowledge as a resource, and the care the patient receives is negotiated. It could be seen as caring about a person. Independence and growth are encouraged.

The learning/teaching process

Traditionally the nurse has 'instructed' the patient to comply with a regimen prescribed by the health professionals. Studies have shown this is not always effective and compliance can be poor. Current thinking highlights the learning process rather than teaching, which means that the nurse 'enables' the patient to change their behaviour in order to manage their condition themselves rather than 'telling' them what to do.

It is not enough to assume that if a patient has been given information or shown how to perform a technique that he will necessarily act upon it or do it, even if he understands why and how. The patient may have the necessary knowledge and skills, but not the required attitude, and his behaviour will not change until he is motivated, perhaps because a problem arises. The benefit of monitoring his blood glucose levels and preventing long term complications may be far outweighed by the disadvantage of having to prick his finger. Admission to hospital as a result of poor control may change his attitude if he hates hospitals more than needles.

Assessment

The patient's learning programme must not only be based on what the nurse thinks the patient needs to learn. Her view will be based on what she knows about diabetes and its consequences, and the knowledge, skills and attitudes she thinks the patient needs to have to control his diabetes. What the patient thinks he needs to learn is influenced by past experiences, existing knowledge, level of anxiety and degree of motivation and it is these areas that she should tackle first. For example, a newly diagnosed patient with an aunt who needed a leg amputation due to diabetic complications, may assume that the same will happen to him, and therefore become excessively anxious and adopt an attitude of denial towards his condition. This will obviously hinder his ability to learn. (A family tree showing diabetic relatives and the progress of their disease may be a useful tool in assessment.)

What are the patient's ideas on health and ill health and how have past experiences affected these ideas?

For example, some diabetics feel well and experience has shown them that the occasional cake does not make them feel unwell. Being told that they should adhere strictly to a diet which does not include cakes in order to prevent ill health does not reflect their own experience.

What is their view of the nurse's role? Do they understand that their education falls into her sphere of responsibility? Are they in awe of her? Seeing her primarily as a figure of authority can hinder learning.

What is the patient's existing level of knowledge? Care must be taken not to assume that a patient understands their disease well because they have had it for a long time.

Direct questions may need to be asked, possibly using a questionnaire, and indirect questions can often be introduced into general conversation.

What level of anxiety is the patient experiencing? Anxiety levels are likely to be higher at diagnosis. The patient may be concerned about the severity of his condition and the effects it will have on his lifestyle, family and future and his self image may be severely altered. Mild anxiety can stimulate the will to learn, but the patient expecting eventually to have a leg amputated, may be too preoccupied to absorb and implement new ideas and principles while others may still be going through the 'grieving' process which could hamper their ability to learn (*see* page 7).

What is the patient's level of motivation? This is difficult to assess, but very important. It can be influenced by feeling or being unwell, by the realization of the potential serious consequences of diabetes or by the involvement and encouragement of family and friends or other diabetics.

Is the patient able to learn? Factors to consider are age, intellectual ability, impairment of sight or hearing or language problems, and the nurse must adapt the learning plan accordingly by incorporating appropriate methods and aids.

To complete the assessment of the patient the nurse should also gather information on the patient's social situation and his psychological state. The patient's job or lack of one, and his housing may be very relevant when considering his motivation to achieve good diabetic control. If, for example, he has just lost his job and is consequently concerned about how to pay the mortgage, it is not likely that his diabetes is high on his list of priorities. Losing the job may also cause him to feel a loss of self esteem. The stress involved may give rise to poorer diabetic control and consequently a feeling of being 'under par' which may make coping with all of these problems more difficult. It is also important to find out what the job is; shift workers may have difficulties managing their diabetes around their jobs for example.

Recreational activities such as hobbies, exercise or involvement in the community are important as they may be very relevant when devising a learning or nursing plan.

The patient's relationships are also important as they can be either a source of support or of stress. The nurse needs to know how well the patient has accepted his condition and what his support and coping systems are. Other relevant factors are what the patient's hopes and aspirations are, and his fears about how his diabetes may affect these. When planning care, it is important that the goals are realistic. If a patient is anxious, for example, it may not be realistic or even desirable for the patient's anxiety to be totally resolved. Anxiety is a normal response in many situations and can also act as a motivating factor. The goal in this situation may be that the patient feels able to discuss his anxieties with the nurse when he wishes. The nurse would help this patient by being supportive psychologically. The nurse, when implementing the care, will need to use her practical skills and those of communication and counselling, and should ensure that she evaluates the care given.

Developing the learning/teaching plan

The aim of diabetes education is to enable the individual to become self caring and so it may be helpful to express the patient's learning needs as deficits in self care as it helps to focus on the learning objectives.

For example, Joan Brown is a 45-year-old woman who has recently started taking glibenclamide to control her diabetes. Following assessment it is discovered that although Joan knows the importance of taking the tablets and knows how they work, she thought she should take them after rather than before meals. Joan's learning need or self care deficit is that she is unable to take her tablets correctly because of lack of knowledge.

Developing the learning plan should be done by the nurse and the patient together. The first objective is for the patient to learn the things that concern him most or that he needs to know to survive. These are often referred to as a 'survival package' and can be seen as making the best of an existing problem. For the newly diagnosed NIDD this may be a brief explanation of what diabetes is, how it might affect him and basic dietary principles. The newly diagnosed IDD will need to learn about monitoring, insulin injections, what to do when ill, driving, basic dietary principles and how to avoid hypo- and hyperglycaemia.

The next stage of the plan involves the acquisition of knowledge, skills and attitudes to prevent the situation worsening. This may include how to achieve good blood glucose control.

The final stage involves the knowledge, skills and attitudes required to prevent future complications. In a young, newly diagnosed patient this would involve learning about foot care. Such information would need to be given earlier to someone with a foot ulcer at diagnosis. This highlights the need to be flexible and to devise a learning plan for each patient as an individual.

There is a great deal to learn and it will take a long time. The patient's motivation to learn will wane as the disease becomes better controlled and when this happens it is more difficult to motivate patients to learn about and take preventive measures.

Behavioural objectives

The aim of educating the diabetic patient is to effect a change in their behaviour. It therefore makes sense to devise an individualized learning plan for each patient which is expressed in terms of behavioural objectives. These should be clear and precise and stated in such a way that the eventual desired outcome is measurable or observable. An example of a behavioural objective is: patient X will be able to draw up and give his insulin injection unaided, using a disposable syringe, safely and accurately by the end of the session. If objectives are written in this way there is no ambiguity, and they are explicit for both the educator and the learner. It is also easier to ensure that the objectives are realistic, achievable, desirable, measurable and above all agreed with the patient. Behavioural objectives, to be most useful, should contain five elements. These are: who is to demonstrate the desired behaviour; what the actual behaviour will be; any relevant conditions that may be applicable; how well the behaviour is to be performed and by when the behaviour will be achieved. To make it easier for the patient to achieve the objective, it may be broken down into stages or small steps enabling the patient to proceed at his own pace and be encouraged at each stage to go further.

Implementing the learning/teaching plan

- Information should be given in stages – clearly, concisely, logically
- Adjust rate at which information is given for each patient
- Patient's understanding should be verified before proceeding to next stage
- Patient should be encouraged to ask questions when they occur to him
- Use analogies which the patient will understand
- Use diagrams, pictures etc to reinforce the message where appropriate
- Avoid jargon and keep medical terminology simple
- Consider language used particularly with patients for whom English is not their first language

- Demonstrate techniques slowly allowing time for patient to practise each stage and with explanations of why they are done in a particular way
- Specific times need to be set aside for teaching
- Informal and comfortable area

On page 28 are extracts from an education plan. These are not comprehensive and should be adapted to each individual. Learning needs are expressed as self care deficits and relate to a lack of knowledge. Learning needs relating to lack of skill or a physical deficit should be incorporated accordingly.

Sometimes the nurse will have subjects she knows she must teach but the patient will not be motivated to learn them. The nurse then needs to tell the patient that these subjects need to be explored when he is ready, and be prepared to respond to cues from the patient. Involving a friend or relative can be helpful if they use their influence.

The plan needs to be executed in a number of stages and each stage recorded.

Dates – when nurse and patient expect to complete each stage and when each stage is actually completed

Teaching – nurse shows and informs patient

Guiding – patient performs task with nurse talking him through it

Supporting – patient performs task with nurse providing psychological support

Self care – date when patient performs task with no help

See illustrations on page 28.

Group teaching

- Can be as effective and more efficient than one-to-one
- Maximum of eight in group
- Learning objectives should be similar
- Individuals learn from others' experiences

Resources

- The main resource needed is the nurse and her knowledge, skills and attitudes in diabetes and educational techniques. Help and support can also be sought from other health professionals
- Literature and materials from the BDA, commercial companies, diabetes specialist nurse, dietician, etc.

Self care deficit: Unable to say what diabetes is and how high blood sugar levels affect the body, due to lack of knowledge.
Objectives: Will be able to accurately describe the basic symptoms of high blood sugar and why they occur, to the nurse when asked.

Guideline	Teaching	Guiding	Supporting	Self-care	Additional information
Where blood sugar comes from					Uninterrupted care
Need for insulin					One to one teaching
What a normal blood sugar level is					Allow opportunities to ask questions
Lethargy					Give leaflets as appropriate
Polyuria and Polydipsia					
Weight loss					
Honeymoon period					

Self care deficit: Does not know the action of his or her insulin/s, due to lack of knowledge.
Objectives: Will be able to accurately state the lengths of action of the insulin/s being used and when to take them, when asked by the nurse.

Guideline	Teaching	Guiding	Supporting	Self-care	Additional information
Type of insulin, eg Long/short acting or mixed					Uninterrupted care
Action - peak, length					One to one teaching
When to take insulin					Give leaflets as appropriate
Relationship to food intake					

Fig. 5.1 Examples of education plans.

Evaluation of the learning/teaching plan

Evaluation of the learning programme is important in showing whether the teaching has been effective. There are a number of ways of evaluating it.

- Ask patient to demonstrate techniques/explain what he has been taught in his own words
- Ask patient for feedback on pace, content, presentation of information
- Observe for changes in behaviour
- Observe for increased motivation and interest
- Observe degree of metabolic control

The nurse's evaluation of progress may lead to further assessment and planning and then further implementation and evaluation with the learning process continuing for years.

What does the patient need to know?

Some policies may vary between Districts and should be checked.

All diabetics

- what is IDDM/NIDDM
  - assess existing knowledge
  - give appropriate literature
  - give patient time to ask questions
  - explain what the implications of having diabetes are
- prescription exemption
- driving and insurance
  - patient must notify DVLC and the GP may be asked to fill in forms with details of treatment and stability
  - licence will need to be renewed every 3 years

  patients will not be able to drive if they have:
  - serious eyesight problems or severe loss of sensation in limbs
  - difficulty in recognizing early symptoms of hypoglycaemia which may affect judgement
  - they are being stabilized on insulin (until stabilization is complete)

  for patients with, or hoping to obtain a PSV or HGV licence, the BDA can provide information and advice
  - patients should always carry fast acting carbohydrate in the car and if possible drive after eating

  At the first sign of hypoglycaemia the diabetic driver should stop the car, take carbohydrate and leave the driving seat until the symptoms disappear. This is important as they can be charged with driving under the influence of drugs without due care if they remain in the driving seat

- insurance
  – patients must inform their motor insurance company about their diabetes. The GP may be asked to fill in a form and the premium will probably be increased

Full details of driving and insurance regulations can be obtained from the BDA.

- identification bracelet
  – it is advisable to carry a card showing name, address and details of insulin or tablet dose, and/or an identification bracelet

- foot care/chiropody (for further details *see* page 70)
  – wash daily with soap and water
  – dry well, especially between toes
  – change socks/stockings daily
  – do not wear tight shoes or socks
  – never walk in bare feet
  – never sit close to fires
  – do not use hot water bottles
  – never use corn plasters or razors
  – see a state registered chiropodist if any problems arise (all diabetic patients are entitled to NHS chiropody)

- what to do when ill
  – never stop insulin or tablets – dose may need be increased
  – perform monitoring more frequently
  – IDDs check for ketones
  – take fluids if unable to eat normally
  – seek medical advice if ketones high or vomiting occurs

- blood monitoring equipment
  – safe disposal of lancets
  – keep adequate supply of monitoring strips
  – keep diary of results up-to-date

- blood monitoring technique (*see* page 17)
  – correct technique
  – correct method of recording
  – correct interpretation of results
  – understand when to test

- exercise (*see* page 43)
  – take extra carbohydrate before exercise or reduce insulin/tablet dose
  – avoid certain activities – scuba diving, high altitude parachuting

- hypoglycaemic attacks
  – signs and symptoms
  – causes and prevention

- always carry glucose
- ensure friends and family know how to cope
- availability of Hypostop and glucagon and how to use it if necessary

- smoking status   Don't! – explain why
- diet (*see* page 34)
- holidays and travel   – monitor regularly
- carry two sets of insulin in two pieces of luggage in case of loss (but not in luggage to be placed in hold of aeroplane)
- take account of time zone changes when planning food and insulin
- in hot climates keep insulin in vacuum flask with cold water
- ensure adequate insurance to return home if problems occur
- ensure immunizations up-to-date
- do not drink tap water
- check availability of sugar-free drinks
- ask for BDA leaflets on individual countries

- job/career   – IDDs cannot join (or sometimes remain in) Armed Forces or Police Force
- sometimes not able to work with machinery or do dangerous jobs, e.g. steeplejack
- shift work – adapt meal times and insulin/tablets to suit timetable

- British Diabetic Association   – all patients and health professionals should be encouraged to join
- provides individual advice service
- publishes bi-monthly magazine 'Balance'
- local branches involved in fund-raising
- organizes holidays
- practice membership available

- contraception   – barrier methods most appropriate
- progesterone only or low oestrogen pills preferable to reduce risk of arterial disease

	– sterilization advisable when family complete
• pregnancy	– pre-pregnancy counselling is essential to reduce the risk of abortion and congenital abnormalities. This involves optimal control for three months prior to conception
	– assess for complications prior to conception
	– NIDDs usually require insulin injections during pregnancy
	– pregnant women should be referred to obstetrician antenatal clinic

Special points for insulin-dependent diabetics

• storage of insulin	– bottle in use at room temperature
	– spare bottles in refrigerator
• storage of syringes	– re-sheath after use
	– store in refrigerator or safe cupboard
	– do not wash
• disposal of syringes	– in sealed can, available on prescription
	– some Districts provide 'Sharps' bins on prescription
• drawing up of insulin	– check technique
	– mixing technique
• injection technique	– injecting at 90°
• injection site	– availability of sites
	– examine for lipodystrophy
	– rotation
• adjustment of insulin doses	– may need to consult GP, diabetes specialist nurse or consultant for advice
• action of insulin	– patient should know length of action of insulins
	– may need to consult GP, diabetes specialist nurse or consultant for advice

CHAPTER 6

Treatment of non-insulin-dependent diabetes

THE primary objectives of treatment are the same for all types of diabetes mellitus.

- To preserve life
- To relieve symptoms
- To improve the quality of life
- To prevent acute and chronic complications
- To avoid excess mortality
- To treat accompanying disorders

Treatment should be tailored to the individual (European NIDDM Policy Group. A Consensus on the Management of NIDDM and WHO Report, Geneva 1985).

As hyperglycaemia causes complications, early detection and control of metabolism are desirable. There are often other disorders and disabilities associated with NIDDM or there may be limited life expectancy. In elderly patients near normal blood glucose control can increase the risk of hypoglycaemia, and normoglycaemia is not always necessary in the elderly with regard to the prevention of complications. Their quality of life can deteriorate with enforced and rigid therapeutic regimens.

Control of hypertension, control of hyperlipidaemia and stopping smoking are just as important for the prevention of complications as blood glucose control.

The impact of untreated or poorly controlled diabetes is:

- decreased quality of life;
- excess mortality;
- acute metabolic complications – hyperosmolar coma (NIDDs)
                                – diabetic ketoacidosis (IDDs)
- hyperlipidaemia;
- chronic complications – macroangiopathy: peripheral vascular disease (PVD) and ischaemic heart disease (IHD)
                        – hypertension, cerebrovascular accident (CVA), cardiac failure

– neuropathy (diabetic foot)
– microangiopathy
– retinopathy, cataract
– renal disease.

Following diagnosis it is advisable to leave overweight patients who do not require insulin on a reducing diet for at least one month. If at the end of this time they have not lost weight, perhaps due to dietary non-compliance, and their fasting blood glucose levels have not reduced, then oral hypoglycaemics should be prescribed. *See* Fig. 6.1 for flow chart on how to assess treatment of NIDDMs.

Diet

The BDA has produced dietary recommendations for diabetics. It is these recommendations and guidelines which should form the basis of dietary advice given to diabetics.

Aims of dietary treatment

1 To achieve near-normal levels of glucose and lipids.
2 To minimize the risk of hypoglycaemia in diabetics treated with insulin and certain hypoglycaemic drugs.
3 To reduce weight if necessary.

Dietary recommendations

Energy intake (calories) must be tailored to individual needs. This is essential for good long term control. The patient should be weighed and the energy intake adjusted accordingly:

- if the patient is overweight total calories should be reduced;
- if the patient is of ideal body weight, current calorie intake should be maintained;
- if the patient is underweight, total calories should be increased in the form of fibre-rich carbohydrate foods.

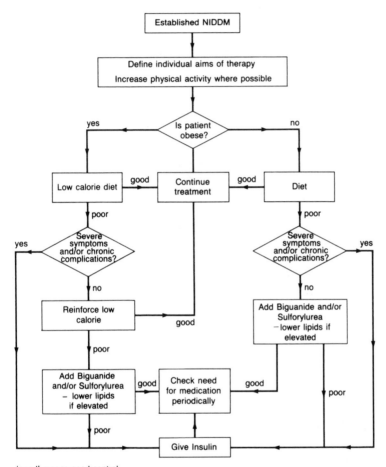

'good' means good control

'poor' means poor control

Figure 6.1 Flow chart for assessment of treatment of NIDDMs.

Carbohydrate

All rapidly-absorbed carbohydrate foods should be avoided

Sugar, glucose, jam, marmalade, lemon curd, honey, syrup, treacle, chocolate spread, condensed milk, chocolate and sweets, sweet pastries and biscuits, sweetened cakes and puddings, jelly, mincemeat, marzipan, tinned fruit in syrup, sugar-coated breakfast cereals, sweetened fizzy drinks and fruit squash are *not* recommended.

Dried fruit such as sultanas, raisins, dates and figs are rich in natural fruit sugar and may be used sparingly to sweeten breakfast cereal or sugar-free cakes and puddings.

Carbohydrate foods which are rich in dietary fibre (*see* below for examples) are more slowly and steadily absorbed. The patient should be encouraged to eat these foods at regular intervals throughout the day.

Fibre-rich carbohydrate foods

Wholemeal bread, wholemeal crispbread, oatcakes, wholemeal biscuits, wholemeal flour, Weetabix, Shredded Wheat, Puffed Wheat, porridge, Branflakes, brown rice, wholemeal pasta, baked beans, potatoes cooked in their skins, dried beans, e.g. butter, haricot and kidney beans.

These foods should provide at least 50% of total calorie intake.

Fruit and vegetables are rich in vitamins and minerals and are essential for good health. The patient should aim to have two servings of each per day.

Fat

The diabetic has an increased risk of arterial disease. The fat content of the diet should be no more than 35% of total calories. The intake of saturated fat (animal fat) should be reduced.

Foods high in saturated fat

Butter, margarine, lard, dripping, suet, cream, cream cheese, cheese, dairy ice-cream, mayonnaise, fatty meat, sausages, salami, paté, pies, pastry, cakes, chocolate and crisps should be avoided.

Use cooking oils and margarine 'high in polyunsaturates' e.g., sunflower, corn, safflower or soya oil. Olive oil is a monounsaturated fat and can also be used. Be wary of unspecified vegetable oil which can be high in *saturated* fat.

All fats are high in calories and should be used sparingly.

Reducing fat intake

1 Grill instead of frying.
2 Cut the visible fat off meat, skin off chicken and skim the fat off cooked dishes.
3 Choose poultry, lean meat or fish instead of fatty meats.
4 Avoid fatty meat products, e.g. sausages, paté, salami, liver sausage, luncheon meat and meat pies.
5 Change from full fat milk to semi-skimmed or better still skimmed milk.
6 Choose medium or low fat cheese, e.g. Edam, Gouda, cottage cheese.
7 Use a low fat spread.
8 Use low fat yoghurt or fromage frais instead of cream in soups, casseroles and desserts.
9 Good choices for sandwich fillings are chicken, turkey, lean ham, tuna fish and sardines in brine.

Protein

The diabetic's requirement for protein is no different from that of the non-diabetic. Certain protein foods have a high fat and energy content.

Choose lower fat protein foods, e.g. chicken, lean red meat, fish, low fat cheese and low fat milk.

Pulses (peas, beans and lentils) contain vegetable protein and are rich in soluble fibre. They can be used in vegetarian dishes and to extend smaller quantities of lean meat and poultry in stews and casseroles. Eggs can be included in the diet – probably no more than four per week is advisable.

Patients should be discouraged from having a cooked breakfast as this will increase the fat content of the diet.

Salt

Diabetics should not have a diet which contains more sodium than consumed by non-diabetics. Less reliance on dairy foods and more on fruit, vegetables and cereals will automatically correct this. Patients should be advised to use less salt in cooking rice, pasta, potatoes and vegetables and to avoid adding salt at the table. Herbs and spices can be used to give extra flavour.

Alcohol

The position of alcohol in the diabetic diet has been reviewed by the BDA (Connor & Marks 1985).

The recommendations are –

1   It is not advisable to take more than three drinks daily on a regular basis. This is a maximum acceptable figure, and it is better to drink less. One drink is taken to mean half a pint of beer, or a single measure of spirits (1/6 gill or 24cc), or one small glass of sherry or wine.

2   Drinks with a high carbohydrate content, e.g. sweet sherries, sweet wines and most liqueurs, should be avoided. If this is done, and if recommendation 1 is observed, the carbohydrate content of the drink need not be counted in the daily carbohydrate allowance. Taste is not a reliable method of assessing carbohydrate content.

3   Mixers, e.g. tonic waters, cordials etc., should have a low carbohydrate content to minimize the risk of reactive hypoglycaemia.

4   If recommendation 1 is observed there is no evidence in favour of low carbohydrate beers, lagers or ciders. Patients should be warned about the high alcohol and calorie content of most such drinks.

5   Food should accompany or follow the consumption of alcohol, but simultaneous ingestion of rapidly absorbed carbohydrate is best avoided.

6   Patients on a weight-reducing diet should take advice from their doctor or dietitian before drinking alcohol. If they do take alcohol the calorie content should be counted in their daily calorie allowance, and should not exceed 10% of total calorie consumption, i.e. one drink daily if on a low energy diet.

7   Alcohol should not be consumed before driving or operating dangerous machinery. The possibility of hypoglycaemia persists for at least four hours after the alcohol has been drunk.

8   Treatment with oral hypoglycaemic agents is not in itself a contraindication of the use of alcohol, provided recommendation 1 is followed. Patients should be warned of the possibility of facial flushing when taking chlorpropamide or other first generation sulphonylureas.

9   Patients found to have hypertriglyceridaemia should be advised to abstain from alcohol for several (two or three) weeks, when the blood test should be repeated.

10 Patients with peripheral neuropathy should be advised that excessive alcohol may aggravate the condition and that they should limit their consumption to a maximum of one drink daily.

11 Conditions which should preclude or limit the use of alcohol (e.g. pancreatitis, peptic ulceration, treatment with certain drugs, some types of liver disease) are as relevant to those with diabetes as to the rest of the population.

Fructose, sorbitol, diabetic products and sweeteners

Special diabetic foods are not a necessary part of the diabetic diet and are expensive. Fructose and sorbitol are the most commonly used sweeteners in these products. They do not contain glucose but do in fact contain the same number of calories as sugar itself. These foods e.g., diabetic jam, marmalade, chocolate and biscuits are just as fattening as their ordinary counterparts. Fructose is about 1½ times as sweet as table sugar. Sorbitol is widely used as a sugar substitute and is about half as sweet as table sugar. Large amounts of sorbitol can cause diarrhoea. Intake of both of these substances should be limited to a total of 50 grams per day but avoided altogether if the patient is following a weight reduction diet.

Acceptable calorie free sweeteners are saccharin, Canderel and Nutrasweet.

Unsweetened tinned fruits, low sugar preserves and low calorie drinks are widely available and can be included in the diet.

Body weight

Many NIDDs are overweight. For these patients the aim is to achieve weight loss and then maintain an ideal body weight (*see* Fig. 6.2). Patients who are overweight should be given dietary advice for weight reduction with emphasis on regular, well-balanced meals.

Weight reduction diet

Most people lose weight very successfully on a 1,000 calorie diet. If this seems too strict, weight loss can be achieved on 1,200 calories and sometimes on 1,500 calories.

Daily eating plan for 1,000 calories
- Milk* –   1 pt skimmed or ¾ pt semi-skimmed
                                          or ½ pt whole milk
- Polyunsaturated margarine – 3 level tsp (15 g/½ oz) or 4 oz per week
  or low fat spread –   6 level tsp or 8 oz per week

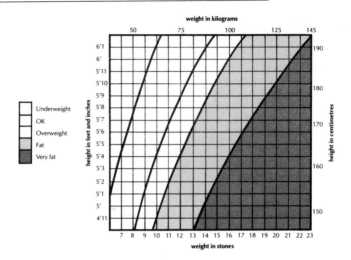

Figure 6.2   Height/weight chart.

Breakfast

- Small glass unsweetened fruit juice or grapefruit segments, fresh or tinned in natural juice
- Wholegrain breakfast cereal, small bowl, or 1 bread exchange
- Wholemeal bread, 1 small slice, or 1 bread exchange
- Milk from allowance for cereal and tea/coffee

Snack meal

- Portion of lean meat, or 1 meat exchange
- Plenty of vegetables or salad
- Wholemeal bread, 2 small slices, or 2 bread exchanges
- Fruit – fresh, stewed or tinned in natural juice

Main meal

- Portion of lean meat, or 1 meat exchange
- Plenty of vegetables or salad
- Potato, 2 egg-sized, or 2 bread exchanges
- Fruit – fresh, stewed or tinned in natural juice

Tea and coffee with milk from allowance, but with no sugar are allowed freely. Low calorie drinks and foods from list on pages 41–42 are also allowed.

*1 small carton of low fat plain or diet fruit yoghurt may be exchanged for half your milk allowance.

For a diet of 1,200 calories. In addition to the 1,000 calorie plan, you may take –

1 extra bread exchange and
1 extra meat exchange

For a diet of 1,500 calories. In addition to the 1,000 calorie plan 3 extra bread exchanges, 1 extra meat exchange, an additional ½ oz of margarine and 1 extra piece of fruit may be taken.
See below for list of meat and bread exchanges.

Meals

Meals should be made up of the foods listed.

Meat exchanges. A meat exchange is one of the following:-

- Meat 60 g/2 oz e.g. ham, beef, pork. Cut off all visible fat
- Poultry 60 g/2 oz chicken or turkey with skin removed
- Offal 60 g/2 oz liver, kidney
- Fish 90 g/3 oz white fish, e.g. cod, plaice, haddock. Not in
                   breadcrumbs or batter
         60 g/2 oz oily fish, e.g. mackerel, trout, herring
         60 g/2 oz tinned fish in brine, tomato sauce or oil (drain off oil)
- Eggs – 2 boil, poach, scramble, omelette (milk from allowance, no
         fat)
- Cheese 30 g/1 oz hard cheese
          45 g/1½ oz Edam, Gouda, Brie, Camembert, Shape, Tendale
          120 g/4 oz cottage, Quark, curd
- Baked beans – 1 small tin (150 g/5 oz)
- Pulses 5 tbsp cooked (120 g/4 oz) e.g. butter/haricot/red/kidney
  beans

Bread exchanges. A bread exchange is one of the following:-

- Wholemeal bread – 1 small slice or ½ bread roll
- Wholemeal cereal – 3 tbsp All Bran/Branflakes/Shreddies/porridge
                      1 Weetabix
                      1 Shredded Wheat
- Potato – 1 egg-sized – boil or bake in skin, or 1 scoop mash
- Brown rice – 2 tbsp cooked
- Wholewheat pasta – 2 tbsp cooked
- Wholewheat crackers/crispbread – 2 e.g. Ryvita, Kracka wheat
- Oatcakes – 1
- Pulses – 2 tbsp cooked

Fruit.   A serving of fruit can be taken as:-

- 1 medium apple, orange, peach, pear
- 1 small banana
- 10 grapes
- 2 tangerines, satsumas
- 2 slices of pineapple
- 120 g/4 oz tinned fruit in natural juice

Other fruits listed below can be eaten freely.

The following foods and drinks are low in calories. Use them in addition to meals or as extra snacks.

Drinks

- Tea and coffee using milk from allowance.
- Clear soup without thickening.

Sugar-free squash and slimline drinks, e.g. One-Cal, Diet Pepsi, tomato juice, mineral water, lemon juice, e.g. PLJ, soda water, Vichy, Evian and Perrier water.

Vegetables.   All salad vegetables and cooked vegetables, i.e. asparagus, aubergine, bamboo shoots, bean sprouts, beetroot, broad beans, broccoli, Brussels sprouts, cabbage, carrots, cauliflower, celeriac, celery, chicory, Chinese leaf, chives, courgettes, cucumber, french beans, runner beans, leeks, lettuce, marrow, mustard and cress, onions, parsnips, peas, peppers, pumpkin, radishes, spinach, spring greens, swede, sweetcorn, tomatoes, turnip, watercress are allowed freely.

Fruit.   Blackcurrants, gooseberries, grapefruit, lemons, loganberries, melons, redcurrants and rhubarb are allowed freely. Fruit should be sweetened with an artificial sweetener, e.g. saccharin, Canderel. Other fruits contain more sugar so should only be eaten as part of the allowance.

Seasoning.   To add flavour to food mustard, vinegar, pepper, Worcester sauce, herbs, spices, unsweetened pickle can be used.

Check list for dietary advice given to non-insulin-dependent diabetics

1 Total calories – body weight
2 Regular meals
3 Avoid rapidly-absorbed carbohydrate foods
4 Eat more fibre-rich carbohydrate foods
5 Cut down on fat
6 Salt
7 Alcohol
8 Fructose, sorbitol, diabetic products and sweeteners

Dietary advice should aim to encourage good eating habits for the whole family.

Exercise

Regular exercise helps to keep weight down and give good diabetic control. Exercise increases the uptake of glucose by exercising muscles thus lowering blood glucose levels. An increase in carbohydrate intake is therefore necessary. The amount of extra carbohydrate required will vary according to the type of exercise. For short bursts of strenuous activity (e.g. running, swimming, football), sugary foods and drinks will be necessary to supply energy immediately and should be eaten before the exercise and after it if necessary.

For more prolonged exercise (walking, golf, gardening) have extra starchy carbohydrate which releases the energy more slowly.

Snack suggestions for strenuous exercise

1 Mars bar, Milky Way, Bounty (mini-size)
4 squares chocolate
1 glass Coca-cola or other sweet drink
1 glass pure fruit juice

Snack suggestions for prolonged activity

2 digestive biscuits
1 fruit with small carton sugar-free yoghurt
1 apple and 1 small packet (40 g, 1½ oz) nuts and raisins
1 bowl cereal with 1 glass skimmed milk

Weight reducing diet case study

Medical history:	Home urine tests often positive
	Blood test at clinic 18 mmol/l
	Always thirsty and lethargic
	High blood pressure – takes Atenolol b.d.
Name:	Mrs Smith
Age:	35 Height: 5'4''
Sex:	Female Weight: 115 kg
Job:	Care Assistant in nursing home
Social circumstances:	Married – no children
Medical treatment:	Metformin TDS

Present eating plan

7.00 a.m.	Tea with ordinary milk. No sugar
	Takes metformin
Goes to work	
8.30 a.m.	2 fried sausages
	1–2 slices bread, white or wholemeal,
	+ margarine
1.30 p.m.	2 slices bread, white or wholemeal, + margarine
Finishes work	+ cheddar cheese/cheese spread/fried bacon
Goes home for lunch	Packet crisps or 2 biscuits
6.00 p.m.	Sandwich – 2 slices bread + meat filling, or baked potato with cheese/meat, or stew + vegetables + 2–3 scoops mashed potato
Daily:	½ pint ordinary milk
Other food:	Picks at crisps, toast, sweets, chocolates, biscuits
Other drinks:	Unsweetened fruit juice, low calorie squash
Alcohol:	Rarely

Dietary advice for Mrs Smith

Energy (calorie) intake/weight

- Weight loss is essential to:
    reduce blood glucose levels
    reduce blood pressure
    reduce risk of other conditions associated with obesity
  This can only be achieved by reducing her energy (calorie) intake.

- Determine a realistic target weight for her height using the chart (*see* page 40).
  - this may come as a shock! If necessary break it down into smaller goals, e.g. 1 stone at a time.
- A reducing diet of 1,000 calories will usually ensure a weight loss of 1–2 lbs per week (*see* page 39).

Timing of meals/snacks

Calories should be spread fairly evenly throughout the day as breakfast, snack meal, main meals.

- Regular meals are advised in order to:
  - Spread the workload on the available supply of insulin. The pancreas will cope better with three small meals than large infrequent meals – improve blood glucose levels.
  - Prevent hypoglycaemic attack – this is not likely with Metformin but diabetics on glibenclamide or chlorpropamide should not miss meals.
  - Encourage a sensible eating pattern.
- Timing of the meals should suit the individual's lifestyle, but to be fully effective metformin should be taken with the meal, whereas sulphonylureas should be taken 20–30 minutes before the meal.
- Snacks are not necessary for diabetics taking oral hypoglycaemic agents and should be avoided in overweight diabetics, i.e. biscuits are not necessary between meals. This woman does not eat large quantities of food at meals but it is all the 'extras' between that increase her calorie intake.

Carbohydrates

- All concentrated sugary foods and drinks should be avoided. They are high in calories and increase blood glucose levels.
- Unsweetened or pure fruit juices are NOT sugar-free and one small glass (100 ml) contains 50 calories. They should be avoided except for 1 small glass daily with food. Diabetic or low calorie soft drinks containing saccharin or Nutrasweet artificial sweeteners are allowed freely.
  Remember that an undiagnosed or poorly controlled diabetic is usually very thirsty, therefore check that all drinks are sugar-free.

- Fruit that is fresh/stewed/baked or tinned in natural juices also contains natural sugars but the sugar is released more slowly into the blood than fruit juice. It is also filling and low in calories. Mrs Smith should eat at least 2–3 portions of fruit daily as a dessert or, if very hungry, between meals instead of crisps, chocolates or biscuits.

Fibre

Mrs Smith's fibre intake is low. Encourage her to eat more fibre rich foods because they help to improve diabetic control, are lower in calories and are more filling and therefore she is less likely to feel hungry between meals.

She can increase her fibre intake by using wholemeal bread, wholegrain breakfast cereals (Branflakes, Weetabix, Team, Fruit 'n' Fibre, All Bran, porridge), wholewheat pasta, brown rice, wholewheat crispbread, potatoes boiled or baked in their skins. She should also eat more vegetables and salads as these are allowed freely and eat more fruit – 2 to 3 portions per day.

Fat

Mrs Smith's fat intake is high. Wherever possible fat intake should be reduced in all diabetics because it is a very concentrated energy source and gives twice as many calories as protein or carbohydrate, and there is a higher risk of heart disease (she is already at greater risk because of diabetes, high blood pressure and obesity).

She can reduce the fat content in various ways.

- Change from ordinary to semi-skimmed or skimmed milk
- Use low-fat spread instead of butter or margarine as this has half the calories
- Avoid cooking with fat or oil, i.e. grill, bake, steam, casserole
- Avoid fatty meats and meat products, i.e. luncheon meat, meat pies, sausages
- Choose lower fat meat (chicken, lean beef) removing any visible fat or skin. Encourage more fish, tinned or cooked without batter/bread-crumbs
- Use medium and low fat cheeses (Edam, Gouda, cottage, curd) instead of hard cheeses (Cheddar, Stilton)
- Eat only two small helpings meat/fish/eggs/cheese daily as part of snack meal and cooked meal, i.e. avoid cooked breakfast
- Avoid high fat snacks, especially biscuits, crisps, nuts

Alcohol

- High in calories and should be avoided except for special occasions
- Diabetic beer/lager is not suitable because it is just as high in calories
- Use a sugar free mixer to dilute

Diabetic foods

Do not recommend them as they contain fructose or sorbitol which have just as many calories as sugar so are unsuitable for the overweight. Calorie free artificial sweeteners (saccharin, Canderel, Nutrasweet) may be useful added to drinks, or as a liquid in cooking, e.g. stewed fruit.

Practical help

Give written advice, i.e. diet sheet (*see* diet plans on pages 39–42). Avoid simply handing out diet sheets without any discussion about eating habits and the principles of how to lose weight.

A target weight should be established and arrangements made for regular weight checks at home and at the clinic. Record data with other diabetic monitoring information.

Congratulate the patient's successes and discuss problems and failures. Remember it may take several months (even years) to reach ideal body weight. Birthdays and holidays etc. may cause minor hiccups but afterwards it is important to remind the patient to get back on the diet and not give up. Motivation is the key to success. Continue to emphasize why weight loss is necessary. Support from the whole primary health care team, friends and family is very important.

A suitable form of exercise should be recommended, e.g. walking, swimming, skipping, aerobics. Referral to a dietician may be necessary if Mrs Smith fails to lose weight or you feel the situation needs more advice than you can give.

Oral hypoglycaemic agents

The patient with normal body weight may need tablets to achieve good glycaemic control.

Oral hypoglycaemic agents fall into two groups, the sulphonylureas and the biguanides (only one of the latter – metformin – is currently available). The sulphonylureas act by stimulating pancreatic production of insulin and possibly increasing the number of insulin receptors on the cells. They are, therefore, effective only when the patient retains some residual pancreatic beta-cell activity. Metformin is used when dieting and the sulphonylureas have failed to control the diabetes, especially in the obese. It is not interchangeable with the sulphonylureas. It is only effective in patients with functioning pancreatic islet cells and acts by decreasing gluconeogenesis, stimulating peripheral glucose metabolism and impairing the absorption of glucose from the gastrointestinal tract.

For younger patients, drugs which can be prescribed once daily are appropriate. The elderly should be treated with short acting drugs given several times a day because of their increased risk of hypoglycaemia. Short acting drugs should also be used in patients with impaired renal function as they are unable to excrete long acting drugs sufficiently quickly and the drugs may accumulate.

Sulphonylureas

Sulphonylureas include chlorpropamide (Diabinese, Glymese); gliben-clamide (Calabren, Daonil, Euglucon, Libanil, Malix); gliclazide (Dia-micron); glipizide (Glibenese, Minodiab); gliquidone (Glurenorm); tolazamide (Tolanase); tolbutamide (Glyconon, Rastinon). They differ primarily in their duration of action. They are more potent but have fewer side effects than biguanides.

Chlorpropamide

This is a long acting sulphonylurea and can cause severe hypoglycaemic episodes in the elderly and those with renal dysfunction. It is usually given once daily with breakfast or the first main meal, initially 250 mg increasing to a maximum of 500 mg daily.

Glibenclamide

This is medium acting and is usually given once daily. Initially the dosage is 5 mg daily (2.5 mg in the elderly), increasing as necessary to maximum dose of 15 mg, to be taken with breakfast or 10 mg twice daily.

Gliclazide

This causes less weight gain and less hypoglycaemia than glibenclamide. Initially the dosage is 40 mg – 80 mg, increasing to a maximum single dose of 160 mg, to be taken with breakfast. The maximum daily divided dose is 320 mg.

Tolbutamide

This is short acting and hypoglycaemia is less of a risk to the elderly and those with impaired renal function. There may be problems with patient compliance as it may need to be taken twice or three times daily. The dosage is 0.5 g – 1.5 g, increasing as necessary to maximum dose of 2 g daily. It can be supplied as a single dose with breakfast or in divided doses.

Cautions/contra-indications

Sulphonylureas should not be used during breast feeding, and caution is needed in the elderly and those with impaired renal function. During illness, surgery or pregnancy insulin should be used. Sulphonylureas should not be prescribed for patients in ketoacidosis.

Side-effects

These are usually mild and infrequent. However facial flushing may occur after drinking alcohol when taking chlorpropamide which can be unpleasant and embarrassing for the patient. Chlorpropamide also has an antidiuretic effect which can result in hyponatraemia and fluid retention.

Anorexia, nausea, vomiting, diarrhoea, headache, fever, jaundice have all been reported.

Transient rashes sometimes occur during the first 6–8 weeks of therapy.

Biguanides

Metformin

This is the only one currently available. 500 mg should be taken every eight hours or 850 mg every twelve hours, with or after food. The maximum dosage is 3 g daily in divided doses.

Before using metformin it is important to ensure that there is no hepatic or renal dysfunction as use of the drug carries the risk of lactic acidosis. Careful consideration should be given to its use in the elderly as renal function declines with age.

Side-effects. These include anorexia, nausea, vomiting, diarrhoea (usually transient) and decreased vitamin B_{12} absorption.

Guar gum

This is occasionally used, but causes severe flatulence which is not tolerated by most patients. It probably works by delaying the absorption of carbohydrate from the gastrointestinal tract.

Conclusion

If the diabetes is not well controlled with the maximum dose of an oral hypoglycaemic agent, plus good adherence to diet and weight control, insulin treatment may be required. It is important to remember that in cases where poor control is observed it is possible that the patient is not adhering to their diet regimen or complying with their drug therapy. This situation should be rectified before insulin is prescribed.

CHAPTER 7

Treatment with insulin

Insulin

Insulin is a hormone produced by the beta cells of the islets of Langerhans in the pancreas. All hormones are proteins made of chains of amino acids and the insulin molecule is no exception. It is in fact made of two chains of amino acids which are joined together with bisulphide links (*see* Fig. 7.1). Human insulin differs from pork insulin by one amino acid and from beef insulin by three amino acids. This difference is important because patients are more likely to develop antibodies, and subsequent resistance to insulin from cows than pigs and less likely to develop them if the insulin is 'human'. Insulin is extracted from pig and cattle pancreases and undergoes purification to ensure that no other animal proteins such as pancreatic enzymes are present.

Human insulin

Human insulin is made in two ways: the amino acid that is 'incorrect' in pork insulin is removed form the end of the B chain using an enzyme, and the correct amino acid is substituted thereby making it identical to human insulin. This is known as enzymatically modified pork (emp) insulin. The other way of making human insulin is to use genetic engineering. The plasmid deoxyribonucleic acid (DNA) is removed from the nuclei of *E. coli* bacteria and part of the genetic code removed. This is replaced by a genetic code which programmes the bacteria to 'grow' insulin. This insulin is identical to that produced in humans and is called proinsulin recombinant bacteria insulin (prb).

Soluble or neutral insulin

This is a solution of insulin in water and is short acting. It acts for six to eight hours with varying peak actions depending on the preparation. The onset of action occurs up to half an hour after the injection. This is why insulin should be injected 15 to 30 minutes before a meal, and some human insulins immediately before eating.

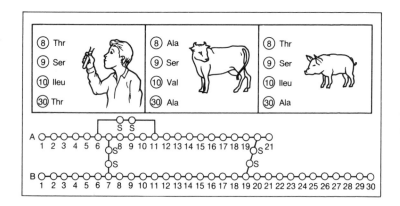

Figure 7.1 The structure of human, beef and pork insulin.

Protamine and zinc insulins

To make insulins longer lasting, protamine and zinc in various forms can be added. Protamine is a protein found in the sperm of the sea trout.

Isophane insulins

These are medium or intermediate acting insulins which have protamine added to them and last for a maximum of 24 hours. Most isophane insulins are given twice daily. They can be mixed in the syringe with short acting insulin because there is no excess protamine to dull the effect of the short acting insulin.

Insulin zinc suspensions

Zinc can be added to insulin in two ways to make it longer acting. The first forms an amorphous insulin zinc suspension, so described because the zinc and insulin combine to make small particles with no visible form. The resultant insulin preparation is an intermediate acting insulin and has approximately 16 hours duration. It is used twice daily.

The second forms a crystalline insulin zinc suspension. This is produced by combining insulin and zinc in a crystal form. As the crystals take a long time to dissolve these suspensions can act for as long as 28 hours or more. These insulins only need to be injected once daily and are classed as long acting.

Most insulin zinc suspensions are a mixture of amorphous and crystalline preparations in a ratio of 30:70; and are usually called *lente*. They have a duration of 22 to 30 hours after injection and are often injected twice daily, although in some patients only a once daily injection is required.

Theoretically, zinc insulins should not be mixed with a short acting insulin, as there is free zinc available which combines with the short acting insulin and dulls its effect. In practice many patients do mix their insulins and as long as their control is good there is no need to change their technique.

Mixtures

There are various neutral and isophane insulin preparations available that are premixed in a vial. These can be very useful for those who cannot manage to draw up two separate insulins, but they may not be suitable for the young who need the flexibility of two insulins to adapt control of their diabetes to the requirements of their lifestyle.

Adjusting insulin doses

Nurses should not adjust insulin doses, or advise patients on how to do so, unless they are competent to undertake this procedure. If the GP and the nurse agree that this is part of the nurse's role, it must be recorded in writing. The nurse will remain accountable for her actions and will be held responsible if any mistakes result from her intervention.

Insulin delivery

Choosing equipment to be used

There are many ways of delivering insulin, but most patients use plastic, disposable syringes which are available on prescription (*see* Fig. 7.2).

Insulin 'pens' are becoming very popular, although at present only a limited number of insulins are available for use in them. The pens are devices where the syringe component and the insulin vial are combined in one system and are consequently easily transportable.

For those with poor eyesight many aids have now been developed. These include magnifiers which can be attached to ordinary syringes and gadgets to ensure that the dose drawn up is accurate. There are also glass and metal syringes available which can be useful, although they require special care in cleaning. The click count syringe has a piston

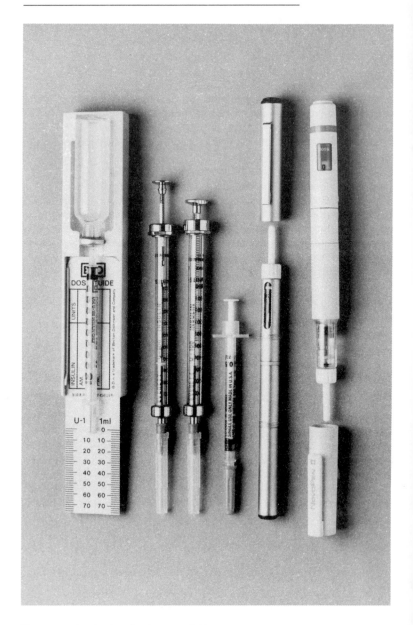

Figure 7.2   A selection of syringes available.

which clicks as it is withdrawn and the patient can count the units of insulin he is drawing up. The preset or block syringe has to be set by a sighted person. The piston has two screws which adjust and lock it in place. Both syringes wear out and must be replaced regularly.

For patients who have problems with injecting themselves there are a number of aids available. These generally work by 'firing' the needle into the skin using a spring loaded device.

Injecting insulin

Insulin injected via a ½ inch 27 gauge needle should be injected at 90° to the skin surface. This is to ensure that the insulin is delivered at the correct depth into the fat under the skin. Most patients have sufficient subcutaneous fat to enable them to do so. Care must be taken with the newly diagnosed IDD who may have lost a lot of fat by the time of diagnosis. In this case the insulin may be injected at 45°. If insulin is given at too shallow an angle, it may be absorbed too rapidly because of the increased number of blood vessels in the skin and the skin itself may be damaged (*see* Fig. 7.3).

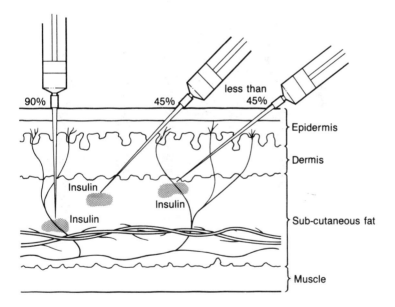

Figure 7.3 Injection technique.

Most patients find injections given at 90° are more comfortable because fewer sensory nerve endings in the skin surface are touched by the needle. It is not necessary to wipe the skin with alcohol swabs before injection. These do not remove the surface bacteria and prolonged use hardens the skin. They can make the injection uncomfortable as alcohol can enter the skin and sting. The skin should be clean and dry.

There are two methods of injecting. The first involves stretching an area of skin before inserting the needle and the second requires a mound of skin to be pinched gently before the needle is inserted. The method chosen depends on the patient's preference. The needle should be held as though it were a pencil and pushed into the skin fairly quickly. The plunger should then be pressed quickly and evenly until it stops. It is not necessary to withdraw the plunger to see if it is in a blood vessel. They are so small in this area that they are likely to be ruptured by the injection of the insulin and an intravenous injection is highly improbable. Waiting for about five seconds before the needle is withdrawn will help to prevent insulin from coming back out of the puncture site. The needle may then be withdrawn; a piece of cotton wool should be available in case any bleeding occurs. This is not dangerous. It is caused by skin capillaries being 'nicked' by the needle as it passes through the skin. This is the cause of any bruising which may appear.

Rotation of injection sites

Insulin can be injected into almost any area of the body where there is sufficient subcutaneous fat and an absence of large superficial veins. Figure 7.4 shows those that are most appropriate. The sites chosen depend on the patient's preference. Insulin is absorbed at different rates from different areas of the body. It is most rapidly absorbed from the abdomen, followed by the arms and then the buttocks and thighs. It is therefore important that one area is used at the same time each day to avoid fluctuating absorption rates and varying degrees of diabetic control. If two or more injections a day are required, different areas may be used at different times of the day. For example, the abdomen may be used in the morning and the thighs in the evening.

It is important to avoid injecting in precisely the same spot every time so as to prevent lipodystrophy. Repeated injections cause the skin to become desensitized, the injections to become less uncomfortable and large pads of hard, lumpy, subcutaneous fat to appear at and around the injection site (lipohypertrophy). Lipoatrophy (unsightly hollows) may also occur, although this is mainly caused by the use of impure insulins. The absorption rate of insulin in these areas is erratic and can lead to

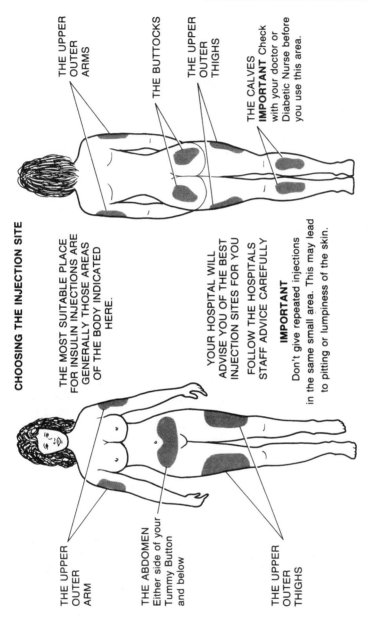

THE UPPER OUTER ARMS

THE BUTTOCKS

THE UPPER OUTER THIGHS

THE CALVES **IMPORTANT** Check with your doctor or Diabetic Nurse before you use this area.

CHOOSING THE INJECTION SITE

THE MOST SUITABLE PLACE FOR INSULIN INJECTIONS ARE GENERALLY THOSE AREAS OF THE BODY INDICATED HERE.

YOUR HOSPITAL WILL ADVISE YOU OF THE BEST INJECTION SITES FOR YOU

FOLLOW THE HOSPITALS STAFF ADVICE CAREFULLY

IMPORTANT
Don't give repeated injections in the same small area. This may lead to pitting or lumpiness of the skin.

THE UPPER OUTER ARM

THE ABDOMEN Either side of your Tummy Button and below

THE UPPER OUTER THIGHS

Figure 7.4 Choosing the injection site.

very poor control with episodes of hypo- and hyperglycaemia. Lipo-dystrophy can also be very unsightly and cause distress, particularly for women. Try to avoid giving an injection in the same square inch for at least a week. A site rotation guide is available to help patients remember the precise spots they have used for injections (*see* Fig. 7.5).

Insulin may be absorbed more rapidly if strenuous exercise is taken immediately after the injection, for example bicycle riding following an injection in the thigh. Hot baths may have the same effect. It is caused by an increase in peripheral perfusion to the area and the subsequent increased absorption rate of the insulin.

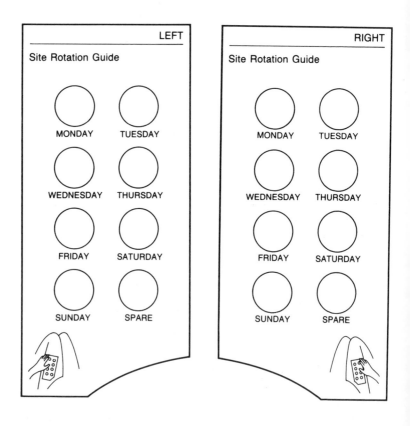

Figure 7.5 Site rotation guide.

Drawing up insulin

To draw up one dose:

- ensure hands are clean;
- check expiry date and type of insulin;
- clean bottle top with soap and water and dry it if dusty or dirty;
- gently rotate bottle to mix insulin, especially if cloudy;
- draw up same amount of air into syringe as amount of insulin to be drawn up;
- with bottle the right way up, insert air into bottle;
- turn bottle upside down, and draw up slightly more insulin than is required;
- tap syringe to release air bubbles so they rise to top of syringe;
- push plunger to expel air bubbles back into bottle. Move plunger to correct mark to obtain exact dose and withdraw needle from bottle.

Remember. It is important that approximately the same amount of air is inserted into the insulin vial as the amount of insulin to be drawn up in order to avoid creating a vacuum which would increase as the insulin was used and could cause problems in drawing up when the vial was nearly empty.

The easiest way to hold a syringe and insulin vial is to hold the barrel of the syringe near the bottom with the thumb and first finger and hold the vial around its neck with the first and second fingers.

To draw up two doses:

- the first three steps as above;
- gently rotate bottles to mix insulin, especially if cloudy;
- draw up same amount of air into syringe as amount of cloudy insulin to be drawn up;
- with bottle the right way up, insert air into cloudy insulin bottle;
- remove needle from cloudy insulin bottle;
- draw up same amount of air into syringe as amount of clear insulin to be drawn up;
- insert air into clear insulin bottle. Leave needle in place;
- turn bottle upside down. Draw up slightly more clear insulin than required;
- tap the syringe to release any air bubbles present so they rise to top of syringe;
- push plunger to expel air bubbles back into bottle. Move plunger to correct mark to obtain exact dose and withdraw needle from bottle;

- insert needle into cloudy insulin bottle. Carefully pull back plunger to measure amount of cloudy insulin. The correct mark will be total of clear and cloudy insulins needed. Withdraw needle from bottle.

If too much cloudy insulin is drawn up accidentally, the whole amount should be discarded and the procedure started again. It should not be returned to the cloudy bottle as some clear insulin will also be injected back into it.

The clear insulin is drawn up first to avoid the possibility of contaminating it with the cloudy insulin. If clear, short acting insulin gets contaminated by one of the insulins containing zinc, the short acting properties will be diminshed as free zinc combines with the short acting insulin (*see* page 53).

Care of equipment

Disposable syringes may be used for up to five injections when used by individuals at home. After each injection, the syringe should be 'pumped' a few times to remove any residual insulin and the cap replaced. The syringe may be kept where the insulin is usually stored. Syringes should be discarded if the needle is bent or accidentally contaminated, or if the markings become indistinct. Some people find that the needle becomes blunt before it has been used five times and they should then use a new one.

Disposal of equipment

Syringes and lancets should be recapped and placed in a 'Sharps' bin or other strong container. A used shampoo bottle or similar is suitable but must be wrapped before being put with other household waste to avoid injuring waste disposal personnel. A needle clipper is available on prescription, but unfortunately leaves a small part of the needle in position.

Storage of insulin

Insulin vials do not need to be kept refrigerated if they are in current use, but they should be kept out of direct sunlight and away from heat. An ideal place in the home is a bathroom cabinet or on a bedside table. Unused insulin vials should be kept in the door or vegetable compartment of the refrigerator. Insulin should never be frozen as this destroys the protein.

It is important to advise patients contemplating travel to be aware of the storage difficulties which might arise. Insulin should be carried in hand luggage and must not be packed in suitcases to be transported in an aeroplane hold as the temperature in the hold may fall to below freezing. In hot countries keeping insulin cool may be a problem; a 'cool' box or vacuum flask may be helpful. The BDA can provide further specific advice on travel.

Dietary advice for insulin-dependent diabetics

The patient should be referred to a dietitian who will formulate a diet according to the insulin regimen. It is important to keep to a regular pattern of meals and snacks. Insulin injections and meals should be at approximately the same time each day with insulin being given 20–30 minutes before each meal.

Hypoglycaemic reactions

These will occur if food is not eaten to cover peak times of insulin activity. A diabetic on insulin must always carry some form of rapidly absorbed carbohydrate, e.g. glucose tablets, dextrosol, sugar lumps to be taken in an emergency.

Illness

During illness the patient may find it difficult to keep to a normal diet. However, insulin must continue to be given. Small amounts of carbohydrate foods in a light or liquid form should be taken frequently (for further details see Chapter 8).

Illness

THERE is a tendency during illness, particularly infectious illness, for blood glucose levels to rise considerably. Certain rules need to be followed to enable the patient to cope with their diabetes safely at home. There might be slight variations in these rules from District to District and the practice nurse should check those that apply locally.

1 Insulin and tablets must never be stopped even if the patient is not eating
2 If blood glucose levels are rising rapidly, the insulin or tablets need to be increased accordingly. Drink non-sugary fluids (sugary fluids exacerbate the high glucose levels)
3 If blood glucose levels are dropping, replace carbohydrate with sugary fluids
4 Test blood glucose levels at least 6-hourly during illness. If the patient is unable to do so alone, arrange for a friend or relative to help
5 If the patient has vomiting and diarrhoea and/or is unable to tolerate fluids, medical help must be sought. Otherwise ketoacidosis/dehydration can develop and the patient will need hospitalization.

Suggestions for carbohydrate snacks during illness:

1/3 pint milk + 1 tablespoon of rice or other dessert cereal
1/3 pint milk + 2 teaspoons custard powder
Small carton ordinary fruit yoghurt
2 tablespoons tinned fruit in syrup + 4 tablespoons evaporated milk
1/3 pint canned soup + 1 small slice bread
1/2 sachet Build Up + 1/4 pint milk
2 scoops or 2 small brickettes of ice cream
Lucozade or Ribena if patient is suffering from vomiting and diarrhoea

CHAPTER 9

Diabetic complications

THE complications which may be the result of poorly controlled diabetes can be extremely serious and distressing for the patient and costly to the National Health Service. Many of the more serious effects of these complications can be avoided, and it is important to ensure that patients understand that the management of diabetes is not only the treatment of the symptoms of hypo- or hyperglycaemia, but the maintenance of good glycaemic control to prevent future complications.

Convincing patients that they should take seriously the risk of these complications is one of the practice nurse's most fundamental but difficult tasks. Patients often think that life is difficult enough coping with diabetes without thinking that it can get worse. They may feel well at present and prefer to live from day to day.

Hypoglycaemia

It is essential that patients understand the signs, symptoms and causes of hypoglycaemia. Friends and family should also know what to do in the event of a hypoglycaemic episode. Often someone close to the patient recognizes an attack before the patient by a glazed look in the eye or a personality change.

A hypoglycaemic attack can be a frightening experience with a feeling of loss of control, which can occur anywhere and at any time. Such attacks are more common in the insulin-dependent diabetic but can be caused by taking sulphonylureas without eating, taking them in over-dose or with co-existing renal failure, hot weather, doing an unusual amount of exercise, taking a large amount of alcohol, delaying meals or not eating enough carbohydrate.

Symptoms and signs

The symptoms experienced are caused by neuroglycopenia (lack of blood glucose to the brain) and the adrenergic response (release of adrenaline in response to low blood glucose). The symptoms may change as the patient ages. Younger patients often have plenty of warning whereas the elderly, especially those with autonomic neuropathy, may experience very few symptoms and even be unaware of a hypoglycaemic attack. The symptoms may include:

- weakness;
- lethargy/drowsiness/inability to wake up;
- tremor;
- paraesthesia/tingling around mouth and in finger tips;
- double vision;
- lack of concentration;
- hunger;
- headache;
- rapid pulse/pounding heart.

The signs are:

- pallor;
- excessive sweating;
- aggressive/unusual behaviour/irritability;
- slurred speech.

When blood glucose drops below normal levels, adrenaline, glucagon and corticosteroids are released. Gluconeogenesis takes place whereby the liver produces glucose which is released into the bloodstream. This tends to correct the low sugar level and may even rebound leading to hyperglycaemia. For this reason it is important not to 'over treat' a hypoglycaemic patient, even though they may be feeling extremely hungry.

At night the patient may experience frequent nightmares and early morning headaches.

Action

Patients should carry emergency fast acting carbohydrate with them. For mild symptoms and levels of 2–3 mmol/l they should take 10 g carbohydrate (3 glucose tablets, 2 tbsp Lucozade, 2 tsp sugar in a drink). If symptoms persist afer 10 minutes take a further 10 g. If the level is less than 2.5 mmol/l and a meal is not due to be eaten they should take 20 g carbohydrate.

Hypostop, which is a dextrose gel, is usually available on prescription. It can be used to squirt glucose into the mouth when the patient is unable to eat or drink, but not unconscious. It tastes very sweet and unpleasant and the patient may immediately spit it out.

If patients are unable to take oral carbohydrate, 0.5–1 mg glucagon should be given by intramuscular, intravenous or subcutaneous injection. If necessary repeat the dose after 10 minutes.

Comatose patients or those who do not respond to oral carbohydrate or glucagon should be given 20–50 ml of 50% dextrose by intravenous injection.

Ketoacidosis

The body cannot use glucose as a fuel so it uses fat and protein stores to provide energy, which results in rapid weight loss, partly due to a reduction in body fat and partly due to loss of muscle. The breakdown products from burning fat for energy are substances called ketone bodies. Ketones cause the pH of the blood to become acidic, hence the term ketoacidosis. Ketones are excreted via the kidney and when they are present in large quantities, by the respiratory system. Patients in severe ketoacidosis experience shortness of breath and have rapid and laboured breathing which is called Kussmaul's breathing. The breath smells of ketones, often likened to pear drop sweets, but some individuals find the smell difficult to detect.

Glucose absorbed into the bloodstream cannot be utilized by the body's cells due to the lack of insulin, and consequently blood glucose levels rise. In an effort to redress the situation, the kidneys start to filter glucose into the urine as soon as blood glucose levels rise above 10 mmol/l. Glucose acts as a diuretic and large quantities of water are excreted. This makes the individual thirsty and he or she drinks large volumes of fluid. Many people think that they are passing large quantities of urine as a result of the amount of liquid they are drinking, but in fact the reverse is true. Eventually a state of severe dehydration is reached. Vomiting is also a feature of ketoacidosis and this worsens the dehydration.

Electrolytes become depleted as a result of osmotic diuresis; one of the most important being potassium. One of the functions of insulin is to transport potassium into the cell. When there is insufficient insulin available, intracellular potassium is low and extracellular potassium is high, although there is a general depletion of potassium in the body. As soon as rehydration and insulin therapy commence, potassium will be transported into the cells leaving a deficit in the serum. This is dangerous as cardiac arrest can result. The loss of sodium chloride is also important as it may lead to hypotension and circulatory collapse.

Some patients in ketoacidosis also experience abdominal pain.

Causes

These are varied. Some patients have ketoacidosis when their diabetes is diagnosed, but the majority of episodes result from infections, other illnesses or errors in insulin administration.

Concurrent illnesses can cause an increase in the amount of stress hormones (i.e. glucagon, adrenaline, noradrenaline, cortisol and growth hormone) that are released into the circulation. These stress hormones are antagonistic to insulin and cause blood glucose levels to rise. Even if a patient is not eating, they must *never* decrease or omit their insulin when they have a concurrent illness, otherwise ketoacidosis might ensue.

Treatment

Ketoacidosis requires hospital treatment. This involves intravenous rehydration, with potassium added to the fluid regimen initially, and low dose intravenous infusion of insulin or intramuscular injections at hourly intervals. Blood glucose and electrolyte monitoring is done at hourly intervals to assess the metabolic state of the patient. The underlying cause also needs to be treated and the therapy required will be dictated by the age and physical condition of the patient.

Hyperosmolar non-ketotic diabetic coma

This is less common than diabetic ketoacidosis, but its mortality rate is higher at 50%.

It usually affects the elderly NIDD, and is associated with rapid hyperglycaemia and exacerbated by the consumption of sweet drinks. The symptoms are similar to those of diabetic ketoacidosis, although the patient is not ketotic, they will have a high osmolarity and be very dehydrated. Lactic acidosis may follow.

Macrovascular disease, large blood vessel disease/atherosclerosis

Risk factors for developing macrovascular disease include:

- Age
- Smoking
- Hypertension

- Diabetes
- Hyperlipidaemia
- Obesity
- Excessive alcohol

Most of these risk factors also apply to the non-diabetic population. More than 10% of the population in the UK over the age of 50 have serious atherosclerosis. The early detection of these risk factors forms the basis of the growing number of 'MOT' clinics held in many practices.

Patients with diabetes are more susceptible and generally have more extensive macrovascular disease at an earlier age which progresses more rapidly.

People with diabetes are 2–3 times more likely to suffer coronary heart disease than non diabetics, and it is responsible for 30–50% of deaths in diabetics over the age of 40 in industrial countries. (World Health Organisation 1985.)

Presentation

Macrovascular disease presents differently according to the vessel involved.

Coronary artery disease

- angina
- myocardial infarction

Cerebrovascular disease

- transient ischaemic attack
- CVA

Peripheral vascular disease

- intermittent claudication
- lower limb ischaemia – cold feet, poor healing, rest pain, ulcers, gangrene

Pathology

Living endothelial cells are damaged and this results in platelets sticking to subendothelial structures (collagen and elastic fibres) and the aggregation of large numbers of platelets. The damaged endothelium also releases a clotting factor. Platelets release a compound which stimulates smooth muscle proliferation. Blood lipoproteins and insulin may be co-factors in this. Collagen, elastic tissue, cholesterol and lipoproteins gather and a patch of atheroma forms. These may ulcerate and a blood clot forms which eventually occludes the lumen of the vessel.

The influence of diabetes mellitus on the development of *atheroma*:

- increased platelet 'stickiness'
- increased platelet aggregation
- increased growth of smooth muscle cells
- increased serum lipid levels
- increased clotting factor
- decreased ability to remove fibrin clot

Autonomic neuropathy

Aetiology

The theory is that this is caused by segmental demyelination along the axon and may be due to a defect in the Schwann cell or primary disease in the axon. In the early stages the axons are intact allowing remyelination to occur, but in advanced states this is not possible. Chronic raised blood glucose levels alter the metabolism in peripheral nerves and accumulation of excess sorbitol in nervous tissue occurs. Vascular anomalies also occur. Thrombi have been noted in intra- and perineural vessels and there is abnormal platelet behaviour. This nerve deterioration is common in longstanding patients.

Manifestations

Gastrointestinal

- Diarrhoea, usually nocturnal and intermittent
- Oesophageal atony and delayed gastric emptying with dilatation
- Gastroparesis with gastric dilatation, vomiting which can lead to diabetic ketoacidosis and chronic hiccoughs
- Constipation

Bladder atony (neurogenic bladder)

Denervation of the bladder can lead to poor emptying and urinary stasis which can result in urinary tract infections. Retention of urine is another possible problem. A denervated bladder may be enlarged, and can contribute to chronic renal failure due to back flow.

Cardiovascular

Postural hypotension may be defined as a fall in systolic blood pressure of greater than 30 mmHg on standing so it is important to measure blood pressure lying and standing (leaving patient to stand for at least two minutes before taking blood pressure).

Blood pressure may drop after insulin injections but the reason for this is not known.

The vagus nerve of the parasympathetic system is affected, giving rise to:

- persistent tachycardia;
- fixed heart rate;
- inability to increase cardiac output which can lead to syncope;
- hypersensitivity to catecholamines, leading to cardiac arrest or dysrrhythmia;
- loss of angina pain – silent infarct.

Skin

Gustatory sweating is where profuse sweating occurs when food is tasted or even just smelt.

Impotence

The sympathetic nerves responsible for erection and maintenance of the erection are damaged. There may also be a psychosexual and/or drug induced problem, and the cause for impotence must be investigated. Referral may be needed for psychosexual counselling.

Hypoglycaemia unawareness

There is a reduced production of adrenaline and glycogen to glucose conversion in the liver in response to a low blood glucose level, i.e. a failure to recover.

Pupil reactions

Pupil reactions are poor and they remain small. Mononeuritis and mononeuritis multiplex are common in the elderly. The third and fourth ocular motor nerves are often affected. Onset is acute and pain is a common feature. Recovery is gradual over a period of weeks. Peripheral nerves may also be affected: the femoral nerves and the lateral popliteal nerve, the latter producing foot drop.

Diabetic amyotrophy

This affects patients of middle age and the elderly. Muscle wasting and weakness are the main features with the muscles of the pelvic girdle and thighs most commonly affected. The shoulders and arms may also be involved. It is usually a painful condition. There is a slow recovery when good diabetic control is achieved.

Sensory polyneuropathy is discussed in the section on the diabetic foot, but it must be remembered that the hands may also be affected.

Treatment

Good blood glucose control seems to be the best way to avoid neuropathy and control existing painful neuropathy. There is no specific treatment as yet. Drugs such as carbamazepine (Tegretol) or low dose aspirin may be used in painful neuropathy.

Elastic stockings may help with postural hypotension and prevent the patient from suffering uncomfortable dizzy turns when getting up from a lying position.

Codeine helps to reduce bowel motility when intermittent diarrhoea is a problem.

Regular small meals and metoclopramide can help with gustatory sweating and an anticholinergic agent may also help.

The foot in diabetes

One of the most serious complications of diabetes is amputation of the lower limbs. More hospital beds in Britain are occupied by diabetic patients with foot complications than by those with all the other complications of diabetes put together. In Britain it has been estimated that the immediate cost to the NHS for major amputations in patients with diabetes, together with artificial limb fitting, is £13.4 million annually and that each amputation costs in the region of £8,500. Apart from the economic cost the social and personal costs to the patient also have to be considered.

Two major pathologies influence the diabetic foot. These are peripheral vascular disease and peripheral neuropathy and are more commonly found in NIDDs than in IDDs. Often both exist to some degree within the foot, but with one or the other predominating.

Rosenqvist studied the prevalence of diabetic foot disease in an urbanized area of Stockholm. The study showed that in a randomized sample of 742 diabetics, only one third were free of diabetic foot symptoms.

If this is considered together with the prevalence of known diabetics in England (1–2% of the population) the number of patients with diabetic foot-related problems is considerable.

Occlusive arterial disease

Occlusive peripheral vascular disease can affect both large, medium and small vessels giving rise to intermittent claudication, rest pain and ischaemic ulceration. One of the problems with the ischaemic foot is that, because of reduced blood flow to the skin, minor trauma results in ulceration which will not heal, infection often follows and amputation can be the final episode in the sequence of events.

If arterial supply is poor, amputation has to be performed at the nearest patent vessel, so that ulceration on a little toe may mean an amputation at the nearest good vessel, often a below knee amputation.

Skin on the ischaemic foot is thin, dry, cool and hairless. It is also fragile and offers little resistance to trauma, so well fitting footwear is essential to minimize damage. This simple measure can mean the difference between losing a limb or keeping it. All ischaemic lesions must be taken very seriously by both patient and health professional. The pain experienced by a patient with an ischaemic ulcer is usually out of proportion to its appearance.

Peripheral vascular disease

Symptoms

- Absent pulses
- Atrophy of skin, nails and subcutaneous fatty tissue, loss of hair on foot and toes, shiny, thin skin
- Cool to cold feet (hot water bottles often used by patients)
- Intermittent claudication
- Nocturnal pain (disrupts sleep; relief with dependency)
- Rest pain (relief with dependency)
- Ischaemic ulceration characterized by necrotic slough, little callous surrounding lesion and intense pain

- Blanching on elevation (dependent rubor and delayed filling after elevation)
- Acute vascular occlusion (from emboli or thrombi)
- Gangrene

Peripheral circulation can also be impaired by the use of beta-blockers which are commonly used in the treatment of hypertension and angina. It is well worth checking what medication a patient with ischaemia is taking.

Finally, smoking by the patient should be avoided or at least reduced.

Neuropathy

Clinical features

The most common form of diabetic neuropathy is distal symmetrical sensory polyneuropathy. Symptoms appear first in the most distal parts of the extremities and progress proximally in a 'stocking-glove' distribution.

Patients complain of 'numbness', 'cold', or a 'dead' feeling (hypo-aesthesia): some may complain of 'burning' and 'shooting' pains (paraesthesia) which may occur spontaneously or upon contact (e.g. with bedclothes).

Motor denervation of intrinsic foot muscles can lead to clawing or hammered toes, while autonomic neuropathy can lead to lack of the sweating function which causes the epidermis to dehydrate and become prone to fissure formation.

Loss of large sensory and motor fibres diminishes light touch and proprioception, the latter resulting in an 'ataxic gait' and poor balance as well as weakness of intrinsic muscles. The involvement of small fibres reduces pain and temperature perception resulting in repeated injury to insensitive feet.

Patients with insensitive feet endure painless trauma that may be mechanical from footwear, chemical from 'corn cures' or 'corn pads' containing caustic medicaments, or thermal from hot water in baths, showers or hot water bottles or from severe cold weather.

The most important neuropathic factor is the loss of pain for it is this feedback that tells you that something is wrong. Neuropathic feet develop abnormally high pressure areas especially over the plantar surface of the fore foot. Callous and corn formations develop and if not treated, lead to aseptic necrosis and ulceration beneath this hyper-keratinization. Serous fluid tracks to the surface allowing pathogens to enter which cause infection in the soft tissue and, if not noticed early, can lead to deeper bony involvement.

Even when ulceration has been noticed by the patient and treatment sought, preventing the patient from walking on the ulcer will be a problem! Rest is essential for recovery. Despite debridement of callous, wound healing dressings and antibiotic therapy, the patient who walks on a weight bearing ulcer will often be walking towards amputation.

Charcot's foot. This deformity is usually unilateral affecting the tarsal and metatarso-phalangeal joints. Poor sensation allows joints to suffer constant trauma leading to bony joint destruction. The foot may be red, swollen and warm and discomfort may be complained of. With metatarsal joint destruction the foot becomes shorter with a reduction of the longitudinal arch. This deformity leads to obvious foot dysfunction and ulceration over new pressure areas.

The 'at risk' patient

As well as the obvious signs of peripheral neuropathy and ischaemia, the following factors should be noted.

Footwear

Most lesions in a vulnerable foot are precipitated by the result of mechanical trauma, from the foot interacting with the shoe and the ground. Always check that the patient realizes that suitable shoes are required for walking in. Many women's shoes are designed with fashion in mind and are not 'foot shaped'.

Shoes should be of the correct length, width and shape and both feet should be measured in the shop before purchasing shoes. If any structural deformity exists such as clawing or hammering of toes or bunions, shoes should accommodate and not impinge upon these deformities. High heels and slip-on shoes are not suitable for everyday use; lace-up shoes with a heel of moderate height provide better support for the foot.

Many shoes are potentially dangerous because they are 'worn out' and nails, metal shafts and cracked leather become obvious to you but not the person wearing the footwear.

The foot

Shoes and socks/stockings need to be taken off and feet examined. Asking the patient the usual question 'How are your feet?' is not good enough! By simple observation and clinical examination much can be detected.

Nails. The reduced vision and frequent obesity of many diabetic patients make it difficult for them to cut their own nails. If nails are normal, i.e. not deformed through trauma, fungal infection or systemic disease or excessively curved, they should be cut straight across.

If nails have any of the above pathologies then patients should be referred to a state registered chiropodist.

Toes. Clawing and hammering of the toes is more common in patients with diabetes than in the general population, partly due to neuropathy involving nerve damage and small intrinsic muscle imbalance.

Big toes can become triggered or bunions can become exaggerated. The overall result of this is that abnormal loading is taken on the metatarsal heads and angular prominences become the sites for tissue-shoe interaction.

Patients with reduced sensation will ignore this friction and compressive stress until corns, callous, blisters or ulcers appear. The sites of corns and callous of today are often where ulcers will appear in the future.

Interdigital spaces. Interdigital infections may occur without warning through poor foot hygiene and fissuring of the webbing. If toes are crowded together perspiration does not evaporate so easily and provides the ideal environment for fungal and bacterial infections.

Soft corns. Soft corns can often be seen between the toes, usually the fourth and fifth where a knobbly joint of one toe presses and rubs the adjacent toe and being a moist area, the corn becomes macerated. Formation of a corn suggests that shoes are too tight and toes are crowded.

Bunions. A common problem is a bunion or hallux valgus deformity at the metatarso-phalangeal joint where the hallux deviates laterally in relation to the first metatarsal. An exostosis or bony prominence develops over the metatarsal head medially.

Friction from the shoe can cause erosion and ulceration of the skin in that area. A bursa (fluid filled sac) may develop which may become infected or the metatarso-phalangeal joint may become infected leading to osteomyelitis.

As well as the hallux deformity the lesser toe becomes clawed with the second toe often squeezed out of its normal position so that it becomes sub-luxed or dislocated ending up on top of the hallux. Due to its prominence a corn or ulcer may then develop on the dorsum of the second toe. If the second toe is in a hammered position a corn or ulcer may then develop at its apex or over the plantar surface of its metatarso-phalangeal joint.

Tailor's bunion. Named after tailors who sit cross-legged while working, this is a bunionette of the fifth toe often associated with varus deformity of the fifth toe and commonly seen alongside hallux valgus. Again stresses from shoe/foot interaction can lead to erosion of the skin, ulcer formation and secondary infection.

The heel

Often the site of ulceration due to trauma penetration by a sharp object or stresses from footwear or intrinsic damage from bony prominences of the heel bone (calcaneum) with soft tissue. In patients with dry skin, fissures often appear around the heel, opening up cracks to the dermis.

The skin

If there are any corns or callous on the patient's feet, footwear should be examined to check size and shape and try to avoid ulceration occurring.

In diabetes autonomic damage to the normal sweating function can occur, so that cracks or fissures may appear in the epidermis allowing pathogens entry, and infection to take hold.

Often between the toes where crowding and clawing exist, perspiration leads to fungal infection and interdigital fissures, especially if foot hygiene is poor.

Poor circulation will result in poor nutrition giving the epidermis a thin, dry, often shiny appearance and providing little protection against minimal trauma.

Oedema. Where dependent oedema occurs in the leg and foot skin which is thin or dry will not be as elastic as normal and may crack or split, thus providing entry to infection. Remind the patient that shoes that fit in the morning may not fit so well in the evening if dependent oedema is present.

Patient attitude

Remember to ask the patient if there have been any past episodes of foot infection or ulceration; look to see if there have been any amputations of toes. Make sure that the patient has understood any advice about footwear and the implications of improper foot care.

Patient attitude is very important in foot care and if there is a denial of diabetes, a fatalistic view of it or a lack of responsibility towards it then the patient is unlikely to take proper care or pay attention to warnings.

Saving the diabetic foot

Despite current knowledge and good diabetic control, peripheral vascular disease or diabetic neuropathy cannot be prevented. The risk factors can only be reduced. Of all the approaches that can be taken to reduce this risk, patient education is the most important. If the patient can avoid the initial trauma, whether they exhibit neuropathy or ischaemia or a combination of both, the sequence of trauma → ulcer → infection → amputation can be halted.

How to save the diabetic foot

1 Patient education
2 Reduce vascular risk factors such as smoking or lipid levels
3 Improve the circulation where necessary (referral to vascular department if necessary)
4 Make regular foot inspections and assessments of patient's knowledge of disease, self care and footwear
5 Treat foot ulcers by – debridement of callous
                       – use of modern wound dressings
                       – reduction of trauma to ulcer (rest, scotch casts, orthopaedic shoes)
6 Reduce trauma to the vulnerable foot by provision of orthopaedic footwear before ulceration occurs
7 Perform regular skilled chiropody as a preventive measure
8 Teamwork and greater communication among medical disciplines

Patient education

Many diabetic patients have been told by their doctors that if they do not look after their feet they will develop gangrene. Most know of, or see waiting at diabetic clinics, patients who have had amputations. Patients know they must look after their feet but do not know what they are looking out for!

Advice must be adjusted for each patient and a compromise reached. For example, an elderly NIDD patient with poor eyesight may be told not to walk barefoot. Such advice if given to a beach-loving, insulin-dependent teenager may be along the lines 'watch out for sharp objects when barefoot'. Below are a number of instructions which can be given to patients where appropriate.

Patient instructions for care of the feet

1 Both feet should be measured before purchasing shoes. Shoes should be foot shaped, of correct length, depth and width to accommodate any foot deformity and if possible be lace-up.
2 Appropriate footwear should be worn, i.e. sandals should not be worn in winter.
3 Feet should be inspected daily for blisters, cuts etc. A mirror can be helpful for seeing the bottom of the feet. If eyesight is poor, a friend or member of the family can be asked to help check.
4 Wash feet daily drying carefully between toes.
5 Avoid extremes of temperature, test water with an elbow or thermometer before bathing. Avoid hot water bottles and, if feet are cold at night, wear socks.
6 Do not soak feet in water for long periods.
7 Avoid walking barefoot.
8 Do not use corn plasters or strong antiseptics such as iodine.
9 Inspect the insides of shoes for foreign objects, nails, torn linings and rough areas.
10 Cut toe nails straight across. If you cannot cut your own nails, consult a state registered chiropodist.
11 If the skin on the feet is dry, use an emollient cream or baby oil daily. Do not apply between toes.
12 Avoid garters and tight socks. Change socks and stockings daily. Watch out for seams.
13 Do not cut own corn or callous.
14 If a blister or ulcer is noticed, apply a mild antiseptic and dressing and consult the local nurse, doctor or chiropodist. It is important that someone sees it.
15 If corns or callous develop or properly fitting shoes cannot be found consult a local chiropodist for help and advice.
16 Make sure that feet are examined when attending the diabetic clinic.

Wound healing

Where diabetic ulcerations occur it is the patient who requires treatment, not just the ulcer. Factors such as diabetic control and smoking have an influence on wound healing.

Modern wound management requires that appropriate products (for many neither drugs nor dressings) are used at the appropriate stage in healing with practical knowledge of their action and contraindications. New products like hydrogels, hydrocolloids and alginate dressings can provide improved conditions for wound healing if used correctly.

The following factors should be considered:

- Is infection present?
- How big and how deep is the wound? (muscle, bone involvement?)
- Is the site weight-bearing? (if so strike through may occur)
- Is there much exudate?
- At what stage is the wound? (necrotic, sloughy, granulating)
- How often can the wound be redressed?

Heavily calloused ulcers require debridement of callous to facilitate drainage and healthy margins for wound healing. But of all the factors to consider, rest is essential. Many patients with plantar ulceration and neuropathy continue to weight bear. Plaster casts, scotch casts and orthopaedic footwear with high technology foams such as Poron, Cleron and PPT aid weight distribution. Shoes with rockers built into the sole can help with load distribution.

Conclusion

Remember:

- Examine feet on a regular basis
- Create a team approach with good communication between disciplines
- Patients with foot deformities, abnormal high pressure areas and a past history of ulcers and amputations require special shoes with cushioning insoles. Shoes should be of the Tovey/Moss type with soft, thin leather uppers having broad, deep toe areas and able to accommodate insoles of Poron 4000 or similar modern foams which do not 'bottom out'
- The provision of regular, skilled chiropody is essential to aid ulcer healing and prevention of future ulceration
- Educate patients and audit take up and understanding

Diabetic retinopathy

Diabetes mellitus is the most common cause of acquired blindness in those aged between 30 and 65 in the West and there are approximately 8,000 diabetic patients who are registered blind in the United Kingdom.

Reducing the risk of diabetic blindness is an important part of the management of diabetic patients and it is essential to screen them in order to detect and treat problems early.

The longer the duration of the diabetes mellitus the greater the risk of diabetic retinopathy.

The causes of diabetic retinopathy are not fully understood, but they are related to alterations in the retinal capillaries, leading to eventual closure of these vessels. Closure of capillaries causes patches of ischaemia which may promote the development of new vessels which are weak walled and may leak.

Other conditions to which diabetics are prone such as hypertension and retinal vein occlusion will also give rise to retinopathy.

Background retinopathy

This comprises all or any of the following: microaneurysms, small retinal haemorrhages and scattered hard exudates. No treatment is required at this stage, but regular checks should be made for progressive retinopathy which will require treatment.

Microaneurysms

These indicate mild retinopathy and show up as red dots on the retina. Their walls are thin and they can leak.

Hard exudates (dots)

Yellowish-white patches with hard edges which represent area where plasma has leaked into the retina from abnormally permeable blood vessels. They leave fatty deposits.

Retinal haemorrhages (blots)

If the blood leaks deep into the retina the haemorrhage will resemble a blot of blood. A pre-retinal haemorrhage with a visible fluid level usually occurs in more severe forms of retinopathy.

Cotton wool spots

These soft exudates are greyish-white, ill-defined patches which occur due to retinal ischaemia.

Maculopathy

These lesions are similar to those found in background retinopathy, but occur in the macular. They are a cause for concern as sight may be lost. They usually affect non-insulin-dependent diabetics. They are not usually associated with proliferative retinopathy.

Pre-proliferative retinopathy

These patients demonstrate increasing retinal ischaemia, increasing soft exudates (cotton wool spots) and deep haemorrhages. The ischaemia may lead to the formation of new vessels which are fragile, contorted and may leak. They should be closely monitored for signs of proliferative retinopathy.

Proliferative retinopathy

This usually occurs in longstanding insulin-dependent-diabetes. New vessels form and are very prone to haemorrhage. At first they are found on the surface of the retina. They then grow into the vitreous and may haemorrhage. The fibrous tissue associated with the new vessels may pull on the retina causing retinal detachment. Visual loss is likely. Ten to 25% of patients risk severe visual loss in two years and 70% risk severe visual loss in five years.

Treatment

1 Obtain good glycaemic control. Reduce raised blood pressure.
2 Photocoagulation destroys (i) abnormal leaking vessels and reduces oedema of the retina; (ii) abnormal ischaemic areas of retina and therefore causes a regression of new vessels and (iii) abnormal vessels. There are two methods:
   (a) Xenon Arc: white light which burns rather large areas
   (b) Argon laser: green light which causes very small burns. There is less risk of loss of visual field and the technique is very accurate.
3 Vitrectomy: surgical removal of vitreous haemorrhage and fibrous tissue. Retinal re-atttachment may be performed using laser therapy.

Cataract

Cataracts are fairly common in patients with diabetes particularly elderly patients although it is not certain that they develop faster than in the non-diabetic elderly population. They result in visual loss. A juvenile type of cataract may occur in the young diabetic, but is rare. The cataract is bilateral and has a snowflake appearance, probably caused by protein and sorbitol on the lens. There may be rapid loss of vision over a period of weeks. Removal of the cataract may be indicated even in a young person.

A problem which may arise in the management of a diabetic requiring surgery, for removal of a cataract, is that lens implantation can hinder future treatment for retinopathy.

Visual acuity

A deteriorating visual acuity can mean progressive retinopathy. Careful examination of the retina through dilated pupils is essential.

Performing fundoscopies and retinal screening need to be practised regularly for the GP to feel confident about his or her competence to diagnose retinal disease. Many eye hospitals or ophthalmic departments welcome GPs in their outpatient clinics to practise their examination of retinas. Patients who are not examined by the GP or who have progressive retinopathy are seen by the hospital.

If a GP is not carrying out retinal screening it is probably preferable that all eye examinations including those for visual acuity are performed at the hospital. This is because while visual acuity may be normal, peripheral vascular changes may have taken place which can only be detected by retinal examination with well dilated pupils.

If visual acuity is tested in general practice, the practice nurse needs to be aware of the correct conditions required for an accurate result to be obtained.

A Snellen chart is used with a row of graduated letters numbered from top to bottom 60, 36, 24, 18, 12, 9, 6, 5, 4. These numbers show the distance in metres at which a person with normal vision can see each row. For example, 6/6 means the person with normal vision can read the 6th row at 6 metres.

Procedure

1. Stand patient six metres from well lit chart
2. One eye should be covered by a card, not a hand. Check both eyes
3. People who wear distance spectacles should keep them on
4. If a patient cannot read the top letters at six metres he should walk towards the chart until he can identify the top letters. If this is five metres from the chart, this is recorded as a visual acuity of 5/6

5. The last line read is the number recorded
6. If less than 6/6 check with pinhole (pinholes reduce visual defects caused by refraction of the lens).

Hyperglycaemia may cause temporary refractive changes in the lens. These are corrected as the blood glucose level falls.

Patients should be warned not to be tested for new spectacles while blood glucose levels are unstable.

Pupil dilation

The drug of choice for dilation is tropicamide. It gives good dilation and is fairly short acting. If the patient is driving or going back to work, then dilate with phenylephrine and reverse with thymoxamine. Do not dilate with cyclopentolate and reverse with pilocarpine as this can precipitate angle closure glaucoma in susceptible patients.

Frequency of testing

In NIDDM patients visual acuity should be tested at least annually. Some patients may have retinopathy on diagnosis.

IDDM patients are not so much at risk in the first ten years following diagnosis and are less likely to need an annual review. After ten years they should be tested annually.

Information on charts other than the Snellen and alternative tests can be obtained from:

British Standards Institution
2 Park Street
London W1A 2BS
Tel: 01 629 9000

Diabetic nephropathy

Renal disease is present to some degree in one sixth of all people with diabetes and causes or contributes to premature death in 50% of IDDs.

The functional unit of the kidney is the nephron. It consists of a narrow convoluted tubule and a tuft of capillaries referred to as a glomerulus originating from the renal artery, supplied by the afferent arteriol and drained by the efferent arteriol. The wall of the glomerular capillary consists of an inner lining of endothelial cells, a basement membrane and a covering of epithelial cells. The glomerulus wall filters different sized molecules and water. The rate at which the filtrate is formed is known as the glomerular filtration rate (GFR). The normal GFR is 125 ml per minute.

The rate at which the filtrate is filtered varies according to a number of factors. Altered filtrating of molecules will cause a change in the GFR. When the kidney allows albumin into the glomerular filtration this is termed a 'leaky glomerulus'. Measurement of the albumin excretion rate (AER) provides a useful measure of glomerular filtration barrier integrity and the earliest sign of glomerular dysfunction.

Macroalbuminuria

If an Albustix shows intermittent macroalbuminuria further testing is necessary, checking that there is no infection present in the urine. When and if the test becomes repeatedly positive to albumin the Albustix usually shows an albumin level >200–250 mg per 24 hours or 140–174 mcg per minute.

Microalbuminuria

This level is not possible to detect with normal stix tests (i.e. Albustix) as they are not sensitive enough. A urine sample should be sent to the laboratory. There are kits which perform immediate tests but they are costly and time consuming.

	Albustix positive
Normoalbuminuria	−
Microalbuminuria	−
Macroalbuminuria	
intermittent	−
persistent	+

The presence of persistent macroalbuminuria is the most important sign that diabetic nephropathy is present. Microalbuminuria shows that there is dysfunction in the basement membrane.

Pathology

The basement membrane of the glomerulus increases in thickness in relation to the duration of the diabetes. The kidneys become enlarged and initially the GFR increases. Gradually the GFR falls and the kidneys fail. This results in raised blood levels of creatinine and urea.

Treatment

Treatment consists of:

1 Maintaining good glycaemic control is not only helpful whilst a person has diabetic nephropathy, but also in preventing the development of this complication.
2 Blood pressure should be controlled at 130 – 140 systolic and 85 – 90 diastolic. Calcium antagonists such as nifedipine, ACE inhibitors such as captopril or beta blockers can be prescribed.
3 When renal impairment increases protein intake may need to be decreased and any protein eaten should be first class. The amount of protein eaten is taken in relation to the serum creatinine levels.

Screening for diabetic nephropathy

This should be done on initial presentation at the clinic and then annually.

Procedure

1 Patient brings early morning urine and dipstix test for albumin is performed
2 Serum creatinine
3 MSU for microscopy and culture. If positive to growth treat and repeat screening test.

CHAPTER 10

Diabetes in the elderly

Quality of life

When dealing with the elderly person with diabetes the most important goal is to maintain their quality of life as far as possible. Many elderly people have physical problems such as poor eyesight and poor dexterity and trying to draw up insulin or perform blood tests can be difficult for them and lead to feelings of loss of independence, inadequacy and depression.

Opinion varies as to the level of glycaemic control which is necessary and desirable in the elderly diabetic. The elderly are more at risk of developing complications, but many have diabetes for years without developing them. Rigid control is often difficult because of the problems associated with ageing. Therefore, as with all diabetic patients, it is essential to assess and manage each patient as an individual, balancing the advantages and disadvantages of rigid control. The usual strategy is to maintain a level of glycaemic control which ensures that the patient does not have any symptoms of hypo- or hyperglycaemia. This may allow an elderly confused patient to stay on oral hypoglycaemics rather than being treated with insulin. This also obviates the need for a daily visit from the district nurse or greater dependency on relatives.

Hypoglycaemia is a particularly dangerous problem in the elderly because of the added risk of falls and fractures, CVA, hypothermia and their consequences. The risk of developing hypoglycaemia is greater when treated with insulin than with oral hypoglycaemics, reinforcing the advantage of managing elderly patients on these agents if possible.

Diet

Adherence to an appropriate diet should not be forgotten as a management tool, but again it is important to take into account individual circumstances and remember the chief goal of maintaining quality of life. The elderly patient living alone may have few pleasures in life and eating may be one of them. To try to enforce a strict diet may be unkind and unrealistic. One approach is to take a diet history from the patient and adapt it to healthier eating patterns with as little disruption to the patient's lifestyle as possible.

Monitoring

The patient's technique for monitoring should be tested regularly. Problems may be caused by arthritis, tremor, hemiplegia or poor vision.

Injections

Again check technique for safety and accuracy. Aids are available for those who lack dexterity or who have poor eyesight (*see* Appendix 3).

Other problems

It may be many years since the elderly patient was diagnosed as having diabetes, but there are also many elderly people who have had raised blood glucose levels for many years, who have not been diagnosed, but who may have sustained tissue damage. They are vulnerable to the affects of autonomic neuropathy such as postural hypotension, poor bladder emptying leading to urinary tract infections and diarrhoea. The elderly patient may present to the GP with a leg or foot ulcer, to the optometrist with deteriorating eyesight, retinopathy or cataract or be admitted to hospital following a myocardial infarction or with severe hypertension.

Ideally the elderly should be cared for in general practice, but there will be some patients with problems which require shared care with the hospital and others who may have been attending the hospital clinic for years and do not wish to interrupt this routine. If the patient is cared for in a shared care system or only by the hospital, the diabetes specialist nurse/liaison sister plays a valuable role in ensuring that the patient receives consistent, organized care and she provides a link with practice nurse, GP and district nurse.

Not every elderly patient is incapable of managing their diabetes. Many are still very active, motivated and capable of assuming full responsibility for injecting, monitoring and dietary control in order to remain fit throughout their old age.

Assessment of the individual and the setting of realistic goals are of crucial importance in managing the elderly diabetic, as with all diabetic patients, in order to maintain as high a quality of life as possible at all times.

CHAPTER 11

Implementing the management programme

Organizing care of diabetics within general practice

The infrastructure within general practice is well suited to the care of diabetics but there is a wide variation in the standard of care provided and the way in which it is organized. Some practices have no special system of care for diabetics, some have demand-led care which has no formal structure and which research has shown is not a satisfactory way of providing screening and education, while others have established diabetic mini clinics.

The advantages of seeing diabetic patients in general practice are manifold. Careful screening and education can, in the long term, prevent disabling complications. Patients are more likely to attend as there is usually little or no waiting time, less travelling and expense are involved and they build up a good relationship with the nurse and doctor.

The presence of the practice nurse is a major advantage in the seeing of diabetic patients in general practice. She is likely to have background information on the patient's social and family circumstances which can be useful, particularly when helping the patient to modify their lifestyle and attain good diabetic control. She provides a continuing and developing role in education and is often available outside clinic hours if a problem should arise.

Shared care

Some patients will need to be seen at the hospital clinic as well as in their local practice. These include:

- those who are pregnant;
- poorly controlled NIDDs;
- newly diagnosed IDDs;
- those who have progressive complications.

The use of a co-operation card is essential (*see* Appendix 4) for the shared care system to operate effectively. Both hospital and GP clinic understand exactly what treatment and assessment the patient has been given and what stage their education has reached.

Routine surgeries

Some practices see their diabetic patients during normal clinic hours, and this may be preferred by doctors and patients alike. The practice nurse is involved in screening and education and it is often her role to identify those patients who need to be recalled and those who do not attend. The patient will usually come to the surgery about twenty minutes before they are due to see the doctor, to have a session with the practice nurse, during which their blood glucose is tested.

Diabetic mini clinic

Many general practices are setting up special diabetic mini clinics. This is only really viable in practices with more than 20 diabetic patients.

Whichever management system is adopted it is important that regular meetings be held with the hospital consultant and their team to discuss:

- treatment and standard of care;
- further training for the primary health care team;
- education programmes for patients;
- role of the hospital and primary health care teams and how they can work together in a shared care system;
- problems that arise in practice care such as the availability of dietetic advice and chiropody and access to HbA_1 or fructosamine monitoring (for example, in Oxford fructosamine testing is not available for NIDDs).

Support available

Make sure that you know how to contact the following in your area:

- Diabetes Specialist Nurse (*see* page 96)
- Local diabetologist
- Dietician
- Chiropodist
- Ophthalmologist
- Laboratory service

- Local branch of the British Diabetic Association
- Representatives from commercial companies
- District health education department

Starting a diabetic mini clinic

Once the decision has been made to set up a mini clinic, it is essential to involve all members of the practice in deciding how it will be organized and setting a protocol. The role and responsibilities of each member of the practice team should be determined and a method of referring to each other established. Once the clinic is operating, meetings should be held for practice staff to review progress and to make appropriate adjustments in the light of experience.

Organization

How is the clinic going to be organized? Will one doctor see all the diabetics or will each doctor see his own patients? The advantage of one doctor seeing all diabetics is that the doctor will improve his skills and learn from the variety of patients and problems he sees, and that patients will build up a good relationship with the doctor. The main drawback of this method is that the other doctors in the practice run into 'de-skilling' problems. Many doctors do not like to lose contact with their diabetic patients as they fear they will become less knowledgeable about, and less able to manage, diabetes. Some patients would prefer to see their own doctor.

Another suggestion may be for each doctor in the practice to see his own patients. They then all become more skilled in caring for diabetics but this can cause complications for the practice nurse, practice manager or receptionist in administering the clinic.

A third possibility is for the clinic to be set at a certain time each month and for each doctor to take a turn in seeing the patients as is often done in antenatal clinics, but this can lead to lack of continuity of care for the patient.

Appointments system and non-attenders

In a practice population of 3,500, about 36 patients will be diabetic; 24 NIDDs and 12 IDDs. Patients will require approximately 10 minutes with the nurse and 10 – 15 minutes with the doctor. If this is insufficient, a further appointment should be booked. If each patient attends twice a year this adds up to 72 appointments a year. Initially appointments may be made two monthly in order to catch up with assessment, education and annual reviews. Recall dates should be recorded on the computer or card index file to enable non-attenders to be followed up.

As well as seeing the GP and the practice nurse, the patient must see a chiropodist. Organization of the chiropody service will vary from District to District, and the diabetes specialist nurse should be able to help arrange for a chiropodist to visit the practice.

Referral to a dietician is equally essential and again the diabetes specialist nurse will be able to help organize this.

Setting objectives

Objectives need to be established which may include:

- identifying all diabetic patients within the practice;
- introducing the clinic concept to these patients;
- involving patients in the management of their diabetes;
- screening for complications;
- agreeing a protocol for identifying risk factors associated with complications;
- monitoring glucose levels;
- monitoring treatment;
- providing education and support for patients;
- providing a system for coping with crises.

Identifying the diabetic population

One of the most important initial tasks is identifying the diabetic patients in the practice. This will be made much easier if the practice is computerized and, if so, the practice nurse should have access to her own terminal. Once identified, the patient's notes will need to be audited and tagged, a register of diabetics established and a system set up whereby all newly diagnosed patients are added to the register. Relevant information should be recorded on the computer or in a card index system. The sort of information needed is:

- age;
- type of diabetes;
- diabetic state;
- therapeutic measures being taken;
- complications present;
- concurrent medical problems;
- current care provision – hospital, GP, shared care.

Having identified all the diabetic patients they need to be informed about the clinic and the way in which it will operate. This could be done by letter, telephone, through posters and leaflets displayed in the surgery and by enlisting the help of local pharmacists.

Conducting a pilot study

If the practice has a large diabetic population 10 to 15 patients could be selected initially starting with NIDDs only. Through trial and error the problems of a particular practice will be discovered and can be sorted out before enlarging the clinic to include most of the diabetics. An interesting project is to compile a questionnaire to give to patients asking why they think they would benefit from attending a clinic, what they find wrong with the clinic at the hospital, in what ways it could be improved and what they would like to see in a mini clinic. Remember that the purpose of diabetes care in general practice is to provide a service which will satisfy patients' needs, and not to provide a service which feels right to the health professionals but does not satisfy patients' needs.

Co-operation cards and flow charts

The key to success in the clinic is having the appropriate paperwork available. It takes time to work out what is required by the practice, the practice nurse and the doctor. Important items are a co-operation card and a flow chart. It is probably advisable to look at co-operation cards used by other clinics before deciding on a particular one. The diabetes specialist nurse may be able to supply some to experiment with.

The co-operation card and flow chart need to be designed so that information recorded on previous visits about blood pressure, visual acuity, fasting blood glucose etc can be reviewed, and the general trends in the patient's progress seen at a glance. Somewhere on the card it should indicate clearly when the annual review is due.

The co-operation card is particularly useful when the patient is being given shared care between the hospital and the practice clinic and the information needs to be transferred from place to place. The patient looks after their own card. This is good for the patient psychologically as it helps to impress upon them that they are responsible for their own health. General practitioners tend to be quite efficient at filling in details, but hospital doctors often need reminding by the patient. It is useful also for other health professionals who come into contact with the patient, such as the dietician, chiropodist, diabetes specialist nurse, district nurse etc, to have an overview of the state of their disease.

Flow charts are similar to co-operation cards but need to be kept in the clinic notes. There should be a space on them devoted to information on how education is progressing.

Clinical monitoring

The following is a check list of what to do and when to do it:

Initial visit

- complete physical examination;
- weight, blood pressure;
- ECG
- HbA_1 or serum fructosamine (in Oxford District only available for IDDs);
- serum cholesterol and triglycerides;
- urine glucose, protein, ketones, infection, microscopy;
- teach self monitoring;
- search for neuropathy – ankle jerks, knee jerks, pin pricks, vibrations;
- fundoscopy (dilated pupils);
- visual acuity;
- plasma creatinine, electrolytes, glucose;
- dietary advice;
- encourage joining of British Diabetic Association.

1–2 monthly visit. This may be less frequent for well controlled patients.

- continue teaching programme;
- weight;
- post-prandial blood glucose;
- blood pressure.

3 monthly visit. As above plus:

- HbA_1;
- lipids (if elevated);
- urine protein.

Annually

- biochemical tests as for initial visit;
- examinations for complications including:
  macroangiopathy
  foot inspection

peripheral circulation
injection site inspection
fundoscopy (dilated pupils) (*see* note below)
visual acuity
- urine glucose, protein, ketones, microscopy and culture;
- reconsider therapy;
- check self-monitoring technique;
- transfer to specialist if progress unsatisfactory.

On some three or six monthly visits the patient will see only the nurse, especially when test results are normal and the patient is stable. If the nurse does find anything that she is not happy about, she can refer the patient to the doctor. The visit should include a blood glucose measurement, weight check, review of problem areas in education and urinalysis. The patient must see the doctor annually.

Fundoscopies. If the GP does not feel confident enough to perform fundoscopies, then patients can be referred to the local eye hospital or to a local optometrist. On the whole the practice nurse would not perform a fundoscopy although there are a few nurse practitioners who have been specially trained at Moorfields Eye Hospital.

Equipment required

The type and brand of equipment used in each District varies.

- Scales and weight chart (preferably in kilos and pounds)
- Height gauge
- Blood glucose strips for visual reading
- Blood glucose strips/meter
- Finger pricking device
- Test recording books/charts for results of blood/urine monitoring
- Sharps box
- Venepuncture equipment
- Urine testing strips for:
  Glucose   Diastix (Ames)
  Glucose   Diabur-test 5000 (BCL)
  Albumin   Allanstix (Ames) or Albym Test (BCL)
  Ketones   Ketostix (Ames) or Ketor Test (BCL)
  Clinitest are still sometimes used, but they do not store well. Patients have been known to swallow them. Clinistix are only useful for qualitative measurement of glycosuria. Ketodiastix may give inaccurate glycosuria measurement in the presence of ketones.
- Urine specimen bottles

- Snellen chart and pin hole card
- Mydriatic drops (usually Tropicamide 1%, Pilocarpine not required)
- Dark room (for fundoscopy)
- ECG machine
- Pathology request forms
- Record card with flow chart (for patients)
- Appointment book
- Recall sheet or card index for recall
- Audit sheets
- Sphygmomanometer and large cuff
- Diabetes 'labels' or 'tags' for records
- Diabetes information books for patient use
- Stethoscope
- Patella hammer
- Cotton wool
- Tuning fork
- Efficient (preferably halogen) ophthalmoscope

Recall

The majority of patients only need to be recalled every six months. If the patient is experiencing difficulties with any aspect of their disease or needs closer monitoring then the period should be reduced to three to four months. Many elderly patients who are stable can be reviewed annually.

Auditing the clinic

A retrospective audit of diabetics is essential to find out how successful the clinic is. It is advisable to audit two to three years hence as well as the previous two to three years and this will give an idea of progress and whether the clinic has been effective. Here are some suggestions for auditing:

First, look up the total number of diabetics in your practice so that the prevalence can be established, i.e. how many per 100 patients. Look at the proportion of types; those on dietary control, those on oral hypoglycaemic agents, those on insulin.

The next thing to look at is the organization of care. How many of the patients controlled by diet attend the practice or the hospital? Of the diabetics taking oral hypoglycaemics, how many of them attend the practice or hospital? Where do the insulin-dependent patients attend clinics?

Look retrospectively at where the patients were seen. How many were seen in the practice clinic? How many by the district nurse at home? How many attended the hospital? How many were not seen at all? Who had a recent fasting blood glucose recorded in their notes? How many of the patients had smoking recorded on their notes? When were they last seen by the chiropodist? How many are apparently free of complications? How many have retinopathy and have they been seen at the local eye hospital? Who has had laser treatment? How many of them have neuropathy, autonomic neuropathy and how many have nephropathy? How many have foot ulcers? Lastly, note down the patient's last fasting blood glucose recorded in the practice notes. This will be very useful for comparing future fasting blood glucose levels and assessing whether they are improving. Fasting blood glucose levels are a very good marker of the quality of care and education the patient is receiving.

These are just some suggestions for the kind of questions that might be included in the audit at the end of two years.

Points to consider

Sometimes both nurse and doctor are apprehensive about starting a diabetic mini clinic. One reason may be that they feel that they are not knowledgeable enough about the disease. The doctor may be nervous about performing fundoscopies for example, and the nurse may feel inadequate in her ability to educate patients about their disease and about her own fundamental knowledge about diabetes. It is therefore a good idea to contact your local diabetes specialist nurse or facilitator who will be able to help by providing further education and encouragement to overcome any hurdles.

Two of the most important ingredients for a successful mini clinic are enthusiasm and the ability to work together as a team. Diabetes is a multi-system disease and involves many professionals from different fields in its management. Essential knowledge is who to contact, to whom to refer and where to go for help.

Education of the practice staff

The British Diabetic Association has produced a booklet on the minimal educational requirements for those caring for the diabetic patient. One paragraph is devoted to the education facilities available in general practice in which it says 'for patients looked after by the general practitioner organized care and education are essential. This is best achieved by the involvement of practice nurses, staff nurses or health visitors attached to the practice and we would recommend that at least one of these should have some special knowledge of diabetes to ensure that there is a satisfactory educational programme for the diabetics managed within the practice. Training of the nurse would not have to be as sophisticated as that of the specialist nurse, but should be considerably greater than exists at present. When a general practitioner has no practice nurse he should seek the help of the District specialist diabetes nurse or the health visitor'.

The nurse within a mini clinic is a valuable member of the team. Her role should go beyond the task orientated function of doing blood pressure measurement, recording weight, urinalysis and blood glucose monitoring. This format does not allow the nurse to plan and assess care or define nursing goals. These tasks should be brought into a framework with education and defined nursing goals.

The practice nurse who is involved in the running of a diabetic mini clinic needs to ensure that she keeps her knowledge about diabetes up-to-date. The local District diabetes specialist nurse may provide study days. The English National Board provides a 20 day short course (Course 928) for nurses with a specialist interest in diabetes which is a comprehensive look at diabetes and diabetic care. The syllabus covers anatomy and physiology of diabetes, counselling diabetic patients, care of the elderly diabetic patient and care of diabetes in pregnancy. The course is available to all RGNs, midwives and health visitors.

The diabetes specialist nurse

The recommendation is that there should be two diabetes specialist nurses per 200 000 population, but of course this is not always met.

The role of this nurse varies around the country and depends on the needs of each District. She will help facilitate diabetes mini clinics and has an important role in the education of all health professionals involved in the management of diabetics. Her specialist knowledge is gained from being responsible for a clinical caseload of diabetics. She should be used as a resource by the practice.

Diabetic day centres

Several centres already exist and it is envisaged that they will provide education about diabetes in the future. They will allow the community to use the day centre as an educational forum and for referral of their diabetic patients. The diabetic population is continually growing. In the last decade the number of diabetics has increased from one in a hundred to two in a hundred. Ways have to be found of providing an effective service, and diabetic day centres are seen as one of these ways. A diabetic day centre employs staff to provide educational programmes and teach and assess patients. They may have a kitchen where the dietician teaches and can put on cooking displays. There are secretarial staff to help with paperwork and patient notes can be kept there. There is a treatment room and the centre provides a base from where the diabetic liaison sisters and the diabetes specialist nurse work. There may be a diabetes specialist nurse who is hospital unit based and one who is community based.

These day centres are obviously very costly but it is hoped that a health District with such a centre could save money over a decade on the prevention of complications through patient support and education. It is hoped that each District will have one within the next 20 years.

Appendix 1: Example of explanation for patients on what diabetes is, as used at the Radcliffe Infirmary, Oxford

YOU will have explained to the patient most of the signs and symptoms by the end of the session.

Hyperglycaemia, tiredness and lethargy, polyuria, glycosuria, and polydipsia.

Obviously the session needs to be upgraded or downgraded depending on the patients' knowledge and understanding. Make sure you give them time to ask questions, or for you to repeat something if they have not understood.

Draw the following diagram explaining to the patients what each part is.

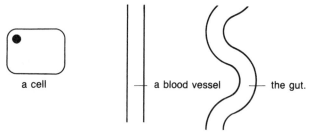

a cell   a blood vessel   the gut.

Draw a 'mars' bar in the gut.

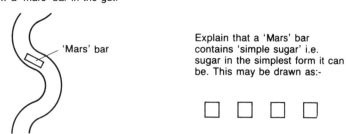

'Mars' bar

Explain that a 'Mars' bar contains 'simple sugar' i.e. sugar in the simplest form it can be. This may be drawn as:-

Explain that these are molecules or particles, depending on the patients' knowledge and understanding. These molecules are absorbed very quickly into the blood stream (draw an arrow to show this).

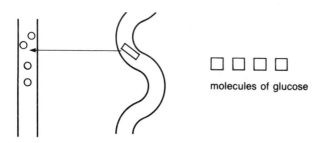

molecules of glucose

Then explain that as the molecules are small they are very quickly absorbed. The absorption rate may be drawn like this.

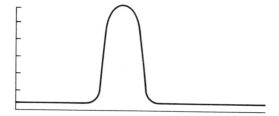

Next draw a potato in the gut. Most people know what starchy foods are but do not realize that they are glucose in a complex form. Explain that the starches are complex sugars joined together with chemical bonds to form a bigger molecule or particle. The molecule may be drawn like this. The whole structure is a complex sugar.

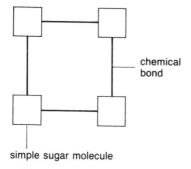

chemical
bond

simple sugar molecule

Explain that before the sugar can be absorbed into the blood stream, the chemical bonds need to be broken in the gut, so making the absorption rate slower and steadier.

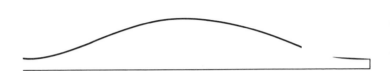

Having been told that they must avoid sugar some people become confused. Explain to them that their bodies need some sugar to use as a fuel for making energy. The reason they are told to avoid 'sugar' is that the simple sugars which taste sweet are very quickly absorbed and that their bodies cannot cope with the rapid absorption rate.

At this point tell them that an organ called the pancreas makes a hormone called insulin and that insulin helps the glucose or sugar in the blood get into the cells. Once in the cells sugar is turned to energy.

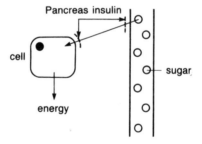

Explain that insulin lets the sugar cross the blood vessel wall and the cell wall to get into the cell where it is turned into energy. If there is no insulin, the sugar has to stay in the blood stream. If the patient has difficulty understanding, a good analogy to use is that of a factory (being a cell) which produces energy. The sugar or glucose is the raw fuel which is in the warehouse (blood stream). If the lorry (insulin) which transports the raw fuel to the factory breaks down the factory cannot make its product (energy).

In the non-insulin-dependent patient the problem is a different one.

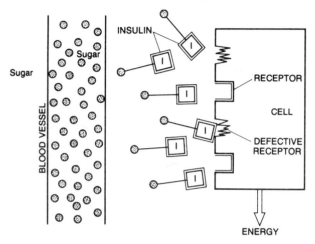

Blood insulin levels can initially be high in NIDDM patients as the pancreas produces extra insulin to compensate for the deficient working of the cell's insulin receptors. Patients who are overweight may have too few of these receptors; in other patients their receptors may not be functioning for some reason. The pancreas therefore increases its production of insulin in an effort to allow the cell to take in sugar, eventually it becomes partially exhausted and stops working to full capacity.

Having explained the function of insulin go back to the drawings of absorption rates.

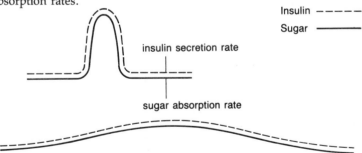

Explain that in a 'normal' person insulin is secreted in response to the type of sugar eaten and that if a rapidly absorbed sugar is taken the insulin rate increases to deal with it. If a more slowly absorbed sugar is eaten, the insulin response is slower.

As a diabetic patient's insulin will be either injected or stimulated by tablets the amount available will be at a fairly steady level, their pancreas being unable to respond to different kinds of sugar being absorbed. Draw a diagram to explain this.

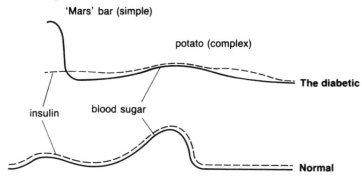

This explains to them the need to avoid the simple quickly absorbed sugars and to eat only the starchy complex sugars.

You may also add that increased fibre will slow down the absorption of glucose from the gut.

At the end of this session the patients should be able to understand the reason for their high blood sugars and their tiredness and lethargy.

To explain the glycosuria, polyuria and polydipsia, the following diagrams are helpful.

Explain that the kidneys filter the blood, and when they recognize that there is too much sugar in the blood they filter some of it out. Using an analogy of the kidney being a dam and the blood sugar levels as being the levels of water behind the dam is useful.

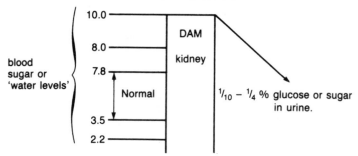

Explain that the kidneys will not filter the sugar out until the blood sugar reaches about 10 mmol/l. The upper limit of normal for blood glucose is 6.5 mmol/l therefore if the patient has urine glucose of 1% the blood sugar will probably be about 15 mmol/l.

This figure of 10 mmol/l is called the renal threshold and may be different for some people.

Explain that as the sugar is filtered out by the kidneys it attracts water therefore more urine is going to be produced.

To compensate for the 'drying out' effect of this the patient will become thirsty and drink more.

If possible follow up the session with something for them to read or look at. Many of the commercial companies produce free booklets which may be given to patients to take home.

To check that they have understood, it is a good idea if they can recap what you have said by telling you what diabetes is.

Appendix 2: Guidelines on standards of safety for nurses dealing with blood samples

EACH practice nurse should contact the local Control of Infection Nurse at the District Hospital for the policy in their area.

It is advisable that all nurses handling blood should have the Hepatitis B vaccination. This should be discussed with the GP.

Good hygiene is important at all times. Risk of infection comes from blood, semen and body fluids, and wearing disposable gloves is recommended while dealing with these specimens. Appropriate safety precautions are aimed at avoiding cuts, punctures and scratches. Try to avoid skin contamination or eye splashing with body fluids. All cuts and abrasions must be covered with waterproof plasters.

Accidental wounds should be treated immediately by:

- encouraging bleeding;
- thoroughly washing under running water;
- covering with waterproof plaster;
- washing eye splashes with clean water or saline wash;
- reporting all accidents immediately to GP.

After insulin injections or venepuncture do not re-sheath or bend or break needle. Dispose in 'Sharps' box. Decant blood into the appropriate bottles and bags for your District.

Spillage of blood and body fluids on surfaces should be mopped up with absorbent tissue or towels and the nurse should wear protective gloves and apron. A bleach solution should be left on the area for 30 minutes and then normal cleaning should take place. Remember bleach can corrode metal and damage fabric.

Appendix 3: Visual aids for diabetics

BLINDNESS or partial sight are not uncommon problems for a practice nurse to encounter. Diabetic patients with poor sight are prominent among those likely to prefer visiting their local general practice to the city hospital and there are also the patients who come under the shared care system. Visual aids are invaluable and a simple device can help someone to become independent in a skill such as injecting insulin or blood testing.

The practice nurse should be familiar with the kinds of aids available and aware of their disadvantages if any:

- Click count syringes
  – patients can draw up air instead of insulin if unpractised, clicks can wear out and become difficult to count
- Pre-set syringes
  – can draw up air and cannot guarantee dispelling all air bubbles
- Insulin pen devices
  – very successful for some younger patients, particularly with the wide range of insulins now available in cartridges
  – can be difficult for the less dextrous to load pens by feel
- Magnifiers
  – very useful, some can also hold the insulin vial and support the syringe and needle thus helping with dexterity and sight problems
- Talking meter
  – expensive, discuss with diabetes specialist nurse
- Syringe/bottle locator – useful

If you require further help or advice concerning visual aids, contact your local diabetes unit or specialist nurse.

Important: It is essential to check monitoring and injecting techniques in patients with failing sight.

Appendix 4: The co-operation card

INITIAL VISIT

		DATE	
HOSPITAL FILE NO.			
DATE OF BIRTH			
WT	BMI	HbA1c	B.P.
URINE	GLUCOSE		
	PROTEIN		
	KETONES		
	CREATININE		
BLOOD	RANDOM BLOOD SUGAR		
OTHER			

		RIGHT	LEFT
FEET	FEM		
PULSES	POP		
	P TIB		
	D PED		
REFLEXES	KNEE		
	ANKLE		
	PLANTAR		
SENSATION	VIB KNEE		
	VIB ANKLE		
	POSN TOE		
	LT TOUCH F T		
CONDITION OF FEET			
EYES	ACUITY		
	FUNDI		
	DILATED		

INSULIN	UNITS AM/PM	
ORAL TREATMENT	YES / NO	YES / NO
DIET:		
OTHER DRUGS		
DOCTORS INITIALS	CIGS/DAY	HYPOS

Review

✔ IF NORMAL ✘ IF ABNORMAL (EXPAND AS NECESSARY) − IF NOT CHECKED

DATE							
WT							
BP LYING STANDING							
HbA1c							
RANDOM BLOOD SUGAR							
FASTING BLOOD SUGAR							
URINE GLUCOSE							
PROTEIN							
KETONES							
CREATININE							
FEET RIGHT							
LEFT							
SEEN CHIROPODIST (✔)							
INSULIN TYPE							
UNITS							
INJECTION SITES							
ORAL TREATMENT							
DIET							
SEEN DIETICIAN (✔)							
NOTES							
DOCTORS INITIALS							

ANNUAL REVIEWS

DATE			DATE		
BP	LYING	STANDING	BP	LYING	STANDING
VA	R	L	VA	R	L
FUNDI	R	L	FUNDI	R	L
PULSES	F P	PT DP	PULSES	F P	PT DP
SENSATION LT	VIB	POSN	SENSATION LT	VIB	POSN
REFLEXES	KJ	AJ	REFLEXES	KJ	AJ
URINE	GLUCOSE	PROTEIN	URINE	GLUCOSE	PROTEIN
	KETONES	CREATININE		KETONES	CREATININE
T4			T4		
LIPIDS			LIPIDS		

DIABETES EDUCATION PROGRAMME

TOPIC	CARE	DATE	DATE	DATE	COMMENTS
WHAT IS DIABETES	EXPLAIN				
	1. THE EFFECT OF INSULIN				
	2. WHY SYMPTOMS OCCUR				
INJECTION TECHNIQUES	TEACH OR CHECK				
	1. DRAWING UP				
	2. MIXING				
	3. STORAGE OF INSULIN				
	4. INJECTION TECHNIQUE				
	5. ROTATION OF SITES				
	6. CARE OF EQUIPMENT				
	7. CAN RELATIVES INJECT				
ORAL HYPO-GLYCAEMIC AGENTS	EXPLAIN				
	1. WHEN TO BE TAKEN				
	2. EFFECT				
	3. POSSIBILITY OF HYPOGLYCAEMIA				
INDIVIDUAL DIET	REFER TO DIETICIAN				
	ADVICE ON				
	1. PRINCIPLES				
	2. REGULAR MEALS				
	3. SNACKS				
	4. EXCHANGES				

DIABETES EDUCATION PROGRAMME

TOPIC	CARE	DATE	DATE	DATE	COMMENTS
	5. DIABETIC FOODS				
	6. ALCOHOL				
	7. EATING OUT				
TESTING	1. COLOUR VISION				
	2. HOW TO OBTAIN MATERIALS				
URINALYSIS	1. TYPE OF EQUIPMENT				
	2. TECHNIQUE				
	3. CAN RELATIVES TEST				
	4. TEST FOR KETONES				
	5. INTERPRETATION				
BLOOD GLUCOSE MONITORING	1. TYPE OF EQUIPMENT				
	2. TECHNIQUE				
	3. CAN RELATIVES TEST				
	4. FINGER PRICKING DEVICE USED				
	5. VISUAL OR METER READING				
	6. INTERPRETATION				

DIABETES EDUCATION PROGRAMME

TOPIC	CARE	DATE	DATE	DATE	COMMENTS
HYPO-GLYCAEMIA	EXPLAIN				
	1. CAUSES				
	2. SIGNS & SYMPTOMS				
	3. PREVENTION				
	4. TREATMENT (GLUCAGON etc)				
KETO-ACIDOSIS	EXPLAIN				
	1. CAUSES				
	2. SIGNS & SYMPTOMS				
	3. PREVENTION				
	4. TREATMENT				
SICKNESS	1. NEVER OMIT INSULIN				
	2. CONVERT EX CHANGES TO FLUIDS				
	3. INCREASE BLOOD/ URINE TESTING				
COMPLICATIONS					
IDENTIFICATION	CARD/TALISMAN				
DRIVING	D.V.L.C.				
INSURANCE	INFORM FIRMS				
FREE SCRIPTS	CERTIFICATE				
CHIROPODY	CARE OF FEET				
B.D.A.					
SMOKING					
CONTRACEPTION					
PREGNANCY					
IMPOTENCE					
TRAVEL					
TYPE OF WORK	SHIFTS				
EXERCISE					

NOTES

Appendix 5: Insulins

Preparation		Manufacturer	Strength i, u/ml	Onset, peak activity and duration of action in hours (approx).
			100	0 4 8 12 16 20 24 28 32 36 / 2 6 10 14 18 22 26 30 34
Neutral Insulin Injection	Neutral	Evans	●	
	Human Actrapid (emp)	Novo	●	
	Human Velosulin (emp)	Nordisk and Wellcome	●	
	Humulin S (prb)	Lilly	●	
	Hypurin Neutral	CP Pharm.	●	
	Velosulin	Nordisk and Wellcome	●	
Biphasic Insulin Injection*	Human Actraphane (emp)	Novo	●	
	Human Initard 50/50 (emp)	Nordisk and Wellcome	●	
	Human Mixtard 30/70 (emp)	Nordisk and Wellcome	●	
	Humulin M1 (prb)	Lilly	●	
	Humulin M2 (prb)	Lilly	●	
	Humulin M3 (prb)	Lilly	●	
	Humulin M4 (prb)	Lilly	●	
	Initard 50/50	Nordisk and Wellcome	●	
	Mixtard 30/70	Nordisk and Wellcome	●	
	Rapitard MC	Novo	●	
Insulin Zinc Suspension (Amorphous)	Semitard MC	Novo	●	
Isophane Insulin Injection	Isophane (NPH)	Evans	●	
	Human Insulatard (emp)	Nordisk and Wellcome	●	
	Human Protaphane (emp)	Novo	●	
	Humulin I (prb)	Lilly	●	
	Hypurin Isophane	CP Pharm.	●	
	Insulatard	Nordisk and Wellcome	●	
Insulin Zinc Suspension (Mixed)	Lente	Evans	●	
	Human Monotard (emp)	Novo	●	
	Humulin Lente (prb)	Lilly	●	
	Hypurin Lente	CP Pharm.	●	
	Lentard MC	Novo	●	
Insulin Zinc Suspension (Crystalline)	Human Ultratard (emp)	Novo	●	
	Humulin Zn (prb)	Lilly	●	
Protamine Zinc Insulin Injection	Hypurin Protamine Zinc	CP Pharm.	●	

(prb) – produced from proinsulin synthesised by bacteria using recombinant DNA technology
(emp) – produced by enzymatic modification of porcine insulin

* Speed of onset is proportional to amount of soluble insulin

Appendix 6: Suggested further reading

General

Bloom A (1989) *A colour atlas of diabetes*, 2nd edn, Wolfe, London.

Daly Heather, Clarke Pat & Field Joy (1988) *Diabetes care: a problem solving approach*. Heinemann, Oxford.

Hill RD (1987) *Diabetes health care: a guide to the provision of health care services*. Chapman & Hall, London.

Kinson J & Nattrass M (1984) *Caring for the diabetic patient*. Churchill Livingstone, Edinburgh.

World Health Organization Study Group (1985) *Diabetes mellitus*. Technical report series 727, WHO, Geneva.

Directory of nurses with a special interest in diabetes, available free of charge from the British Diabetic Association.

Diet

British Diabetic Association (1982) *Dietary recommendations for diabetics for the 1980s*. Human nutrition: applied nutrition 36a, 378–394.

Conner H & Marks V (1985) *Alcohol and diabetes*. A position paper prepared by the Nutrition sub-committee of the British Diabetic Association. Human nutrition: applied nutrition 39a, 393–399.

The British Diabetic Association produces booklets and leaflets on diet.

Nursing process/education

Baksi AK, Hide D & Giles G (1984) *Diabetes education*. John Wiley & Sons, Chichester.

Becker P (1976) *The health belief model in personal health behaviour*. Charles B Slack Co, New Jersey.

Orem D (1985) *Nursing: concepts of practice*. McGraw-Hill, New York.

Pearson A & Vaughn A (1986) *Models for nursing practice*. Heinemann, Oxford.

Stewart W (1983) *Counselling in nursing: a problem solving approach*. Harper & Row, London.

The diabetic foot

Tovey FI (1986) Care of the diabetic foot. *Practical diabetes*, **3**: 13–14.

Index